Exercises For Osteoporosis Book For Seniors

Exercises For Osteoporosis Book For Seniors: Fortify Your Bones, Defend Against Osteoporosis, And Reduce Fracture Risk.

Bonus: 30 Days Exercise Plan For Seniors

ESTHER R. JOHNSON

Copyright

© 2023 [Esther R. Johnson]. All rights reserved. Except for brief quotations included in critical reviews and certain other noncommercial uses allowed by copyright law, no part of this book, "Exercises for Osteoporosis: A Guide for Seniors," might be duplicated, disseminated, or communicated in any structure or using any and all means, including copying, recording, or other electronic or mechanical techniques, without the earlier consent of the creator.

Disclaimer:

This book's exercises and material are meant to be used solely for general educational purposes. They should never be used in place of expert medical advice, diagnosis, or care. When in doubt about a medical problem, never hesitate to consult your doctor or another trained healthcare professional. Any harm, loss, or unfavorable consequence arising directly or indirectly from the use of the exercises or material in this book is disclaimed by the author and publisher. Before beginning any new fitness program, it is imperative to speak with a healthcare provider, particularly if you have any pre-existing medical ailments or concerns.

About the author

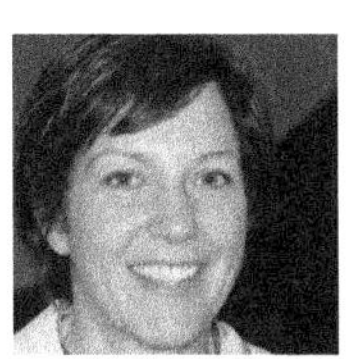 I'm a renowned physician with a focus on managing osteoporosis and geriatrics, Dr. Esther R. Johnson. I have devoted my career to enhancing the well-being of senior citizens and have a wealth of knowledge in the field of senior healthcare. In addition to osteoporosis diagnosis and treatment, I also specialize in holistic elder health, highlighting the critical role physical activity has in preserving general wellness.

As a medical professional in practice, I have seen firsthand the transformational potential of senior-specific exercises, especially those that tackle osteoporosis. My dedication to encouraging healthy aging inspired me to create a thorough manual that combines my expertise in medicine with useful, senior-friendly activities.

I offer a carefully chosen selection of activities in "Exercises for Osteoporosis: A Guide for Seniors," which are designed to improve bone health and general mobility in the elderly. Each exercise has been carefully chosen to be safe, effective, and especially helpful for individuals treating osteoporosis, drawing on my knowledge in medicine.

For seniors looking to proactively maintain their bone health under the supervision of an experienced medical expert, this book is an invaluable resource. My focus on the value of exercise as a therapeutic and preventive tool is a reflection of my commitment to enabling elders to enjoy active, full lives.

By means of this guide, I broaden the scope of my medical knowledge beyond the clinic walls and provide seniors with a useful instrument to adopt a proactive strategy for managing osteoporosis.

BONUS

30 days exercise plan for seniors

ALL EXERCISES IN THIS BOOK

Certainly! Here's a 30-day exercise plan for seniors focusing on balance and stability, flexibility, and range of motion. It's important to consult with a healthcare professional before starting any new exercise routine, especially if you have pre-existing health conditions.

Week 1-2: Balance and Stability

Day 1-3:

- Warm-up: 5 minutes of light cardio (walking in place).

- Balance Exercise: Stand on one leg for 30 seconds, repeat on the other leg. Perform 2 sets.

- Stability Exercise: Chair squats - Sit and stand from a chair without using your hands. Do 2 sets of 10 repetitions.

Day 4-6:

- Warm-up: 5 minutes of light cardio.

- Balance Exercise: Heel-to-toe walk - Walk in a straight line, placing the heel of one foot just in front of the toes of the other. Repeat for 5 minutes.

- Stability Exercise: Wall push-ups - Stand arm's length away from a wall and perform 2 sets of 10 push-ups.

Day 7: Rest Day

Week3-4: Incorporating Tai Chi and Yoga

Day 8-10:

- Warm-up: 5 minutes of light cardio.

- Tai Chi: Follow a beginner's Tai Chi video for 15 minutes.

- Yoga for Stability: Mountain Pose and Tree Pose for 10 minutes.

Day 11-13:

- Warm-up: 5 minutes of light cardio.

- Tai Chi: Continue with a Tai Chi routine.

- Yoga for Stability: Warrior Pose and Chair Pose for 10 minutes.

Day 14: Rest Day

Week5-6: Functional Movements

Day 15-17:

- Warm-up: 5 minutes of light cardio.

- Functional Movement: Practice getting up from a chair without using your hands. Perform 2 sets of 10 repetitions.

- Daily Activities Exercise: Mimic activities like reaching for an item on a high shelf or picking up something from the floor.

Day 18-20:

- Warm-up: 5 minutes of light cardio.

- Functional Movement: Side leg raises while holding onto a sturdy surface. Do 2 sets of 12 on each side.

- Daily Activities Exercise: Practice walking and turning smoothly.

Day 21: Rest Day

Week7-8: Flexibility and Range of Motion

Day 22-24:

- Warm-up: 5 minutes of light cardio.

- Gentle Stretching: Neck stretches, shoulder rolls, and wrist circles. Hold each stretch for 15-30 seconds.

- Yoga for Joint Mobility: Cat-Cow Stretch and Child's Pose for 15 minutes.

Day 25-27:

- Warm-up: 5 minutes of light cardio.

- Pilates for Mobility: Pelvic tilts and ankle circles. Perform 2 sets of 10 repetitions for each exercise.

- Gentle Stretching: Seated forward bends and seated leg stretches.

Day 28: Rest Day

Week9-10: Including Stretching in Daily Routine

Day 29-30:

- Warm-up: 5 minutes of light cardio.

- Full Body Stretch Routine: Incorporate stretches for the neck, shoulders, back, hips, and legs. Hold each stretch for 20-30 seconds.

- Breathing Exercises: Finish with deep breathing exercises for relaxation.

Remember to listen to your body and modify exercises as needed. Gradually progress in intensity and duration as your strength and confidence improve. If you experience pain or discomfort, consult with a healthcare professional.

Table of contents

INTRODUCTION

Thank you for visiting "Strong Bones for Life: A Comprehensive Guide to Osteoporosis Exercises for Seniors." The purpose of this book is to provide seniors with the information and resources they need to improve their bone health by following safe, customized exercise regimens. Osteoporosis, a disorder that affects bone strength and density, can be difficult to manage, but with the correct care, your bone health can be preserved or even improved.

We'll go over the basics of osteoporosis in this tutorial, including its causes, risk factors, and the critical role exercise plays in both treating and preventing the disease. We'll explore a variety of activities designed especially for seniors, taking into account their unique requirements, capabilities, and medical concerns.

Every chapter has been painstakingly written to bring you insightful knowledge and useful advice. This book is your go-to reference for keeping strong and resilient bones—from comprehending the significance of weight-bearing activities and strength training to adding balance, flexibility, and lifestyle modifications.

When you go out on this path to better bone health, keep in mind that safety comes first. Speak with your healthcare provider before starting any exercise program to be sure the exercises are appropriate for you.table for your particular medical condition. While this book serves as a guide, you should work with your healthcare professional to customize these exercises to meet your unique needs.

Let's now go off on a path to healthier bones, enhanced vitality, and a higher standard of living. We'll navigate the world of osteoporosis workouts together so you may take control of your health and get the rewards of leading an active and satisfying life.

CHAPTER 1:

Understanding OsteoporosiS

What is osteoporosis?

Your bones are far brittler and weaker than they should be if you have osteoporosis.

What is osteoporosis?

A disorder called osteoporosis causes your bones to deteriorate. Your bones become less thick and thinner than they should be as a result. Bone fractures, or shattered bones, are far more common in people with osteoporosis.

Generally speaking, your bones are robust and dense enough to sustain your weight and withstand most types of impacts. Your bones' natural capacity to regenerate (remodel) themselves and lose some of their density as you age. Your bones are weaker and far more brittle than they should be if you have osteoporosis. Most patients with osteoporosis know nothing about their condition until they break a bone. Any of your bones could shatter with osteoporosis, however the following are the most frequently affected:

- fractures of the hips.

- wrists.

- vertebral fractures in the spine.

Your chance of suffering from bone fractures decreases with the prompt diagnosis of osteoporosis by a medical professional. See your doctor about having your bone density checked, particularly if you are older than 65, have experienced a bone fracture after the age of 50, or have osteoporosis in your biological family.

Osteoporosis risk factors

An individual can get osteoporosis.

- Anybody over 50 is among the demographics most likely to encounter it.

- Individuals classified as female at birth (AFAB), particularly those who are AFAB after menopause.

- Those with a family history of osteoporosis, if any member of your biological family is affected.
- those with "smaller frames' ' or those who are naturally slim Since they typically have less natural bone mass, people with slimmer statutes may be more affected by any reductions.
- those who consume tobacco goods or smoke.

Osteoporosis can be exacerbated by a number of medical disorders, including:

- Endocrine disorders include any illness that affects the thyroid, parathyroid glands, or hormones (e.g., diabetes, thyroid disease).
- disorders of the digestive system (such as inflammatory bowel disease [IBD] and celiac disease).
- bone-related autoimmune diseases (such as rheumatoid arthritis or ankylosing spondylitis, which is an arthritis affecting the spine).
- Blood diseases (or blood-related malignancies, such as multiple myeloma).

Your chance of developing osteoporosis may be increased by certain drugs or surgical procedures

- Diuretics are drugs that reduce blood pressure and help the body rid itself of excess fluid.
- Corticosteroids, or anti-inflammatory drugs.
- Drugs for the treatment of seizures.
- Bariatric surgery, or losing weight.
- Hormone therapy in the treatment of cancer, particularly prostate and breast cancer.
- Anticoagulants.
- Proton pump inhibitors (such as those used for acid reflux, which may impair the absorption of calcium in the body).

There are several dietary and activity habits that can increase your risk of osteoporosis. These include:

- Inadequate consumption of calcium and vitamin D.
- Not engaging in adequate physical activity.
- Consuming alcohol on a daily basis (more than two drinks).

Management and Treatment

How is osteoporosis treated?

A combination of treatments that slow down bone loss and strengthen your remaining bone tissue will be recommended by your healthcare professional. Preventing bone fractures is crucial while treating osteoporosis.

Among the most popular therapies for osteoporosis are:

- Practice: Frequent exercise helps build stronger bones, as well as stronger muscles, tendons, and ligaments throughout your body. Weight-bearing exercises may be recommended by your healthcare professional to build muscle and improve your balance. Exercises that force your body to fight against gravity, such as tai chi, yoga, Pilates, and walking, can help you become more balanced and strong without overstressing your bones. To discover the exercises and motions that are best for you, you might need to consult with a physical therapist.

- Vitamin and mineral supplements: You may require calcium or vitamin D supplements, either prescribed or purchased over-the-counter. Which type, how often, and what dosage you require will all be determined by your provider.

- Osteoporosis medication: Your physician will advise you on the appropriate medications based on your individual needs. Bisphosphonates and hormone therapy, such as replacement testosterone or estrogen, are among the most often prescribed drugs for osteoporosis. Individuals who have a high risk of fractures or severe osteoporosis may require medicine, such as romosozumab, denosumab, and parathyroid hormone (PTH) analogs. Usually, injections are used to administer these drugs.

Importance of Exercise for Bone Health

Sedentism, unfortunate stance, unfortunate equilibrium, and powerless muscles all add to an expanded gamble of cracks. Exercise can assist individuals with osteoporosis work on their wellbeing in various ways, including:

- Decrease in bone loss
- Increased bone mass
- Preserving the residual bone tissue
- Enhanced physical fitness
- Enhanced muscular strength
- Increased reaction time
- Improved mobility
- Improved balance and coordination
- Lower risk of bone fractures as a result of falls
- Lessened discomfort
- Enhanced mood and vitality.

How common is osteoporosis?

In the United States, more than 50 million people have osteoporosis.

Osteoporosis is frequent in persons over the age of 50. Experts believe that half of all persons born female and one in every four people born male have osteoporosis.

According to studies, one in every three persons over the age of 50 who do not have osteoporosis has some degree of diminished bone density (osteopenia). People suffering from osteopenia show early indicators of osteoporosis. Whenever left untreated, osteopenia can advance to osteoporosis.

Symptoms and Causes

What are osteoporosis symptoms?

Osteoporosis does not have symptoms like many other medical disorders. That is why healthcare experts refer to it as a quiet sickness.

You will not feel or notice anything that indicates you may have osteoporosis. You won't experience a headache, fever, or stomach ache to alert you that something is wrong with your body.

The most typical "symptom" is unexpectedly breaking a bone, especially after a little fall or mishap that would normally not affect you.

Although osteoporosis does not create symptoms, you may notice a few changes in your body that indicate your bones are losing strength or density. These osteoporosis warning signals include:

- You've lost an inch or more of your height.
- Natural posture changes (stooping or bending forward more).
- Shortness of breath (if the disks in your spine are compressed to the point where your lung capacity is reduced).
- Lower back ache (lumbar spine pain).

It may be difficult to detect changes in your own physical appearance. A loved one is more likely to notice changes in your body (particularly in your height or posture). People sometimes make fun of older people "shrinking" as they become older, but this can be an indication that you should see a doctor for a bone density test.

What causes osteoporosis?

Osteoporosis develops as you age and your bones lose their ability to renew and repair.

Your bones, like any other component of your body, are made of living tissue. Although it may not appear so,

they are constantly replenishing their own cells and tissue throughout your life. Until around the age of 30,

24

your body naturally grows more bone than it loses. After the age of 35, bone breakdown happens speedier than your body can fix it, bringing about a consistent reduction of bone mass.

When you have osteoporosis, you lose bone mass more quickly. Postmenopausal women lose bone mass at an even higher rate.

Diagnosis and Tests

How is osteoporosis diagnosed?

A bone density test will be used by a healthcare provider to detect osteoporosis. A bone density test is a type of imaging examination that determines the strength of your bones. It uses X-rays to determine the amount of calcium and other minerals in your bones.

DEXA scans, DXA scans, and bone density scans are all terms used by healthcare providers to describe bone density testing. All of these are distinct names for the same exam.

A bone density test employs low-dose X-rays to determine the density and mineral content of your bones.

It's similar to a standard X-ray. Because it is an outpatient operation, you will not be required to stay in the hospital. You may leave as soon as your test is over. This test contains no needles or injections.

The best technique to detect osteoporosis before it causes a bone fracture is to monitor your bone density. If you have a family history of osteoporosis, are over 50, or have osteopenia, your provider may advise you to have frequent bone density testing.

Prevention

How might I diminish my possibilities creating osteoporosis?

Exercise and getting adequate calcium and vitamin D in your diet are usually enough to keep osteoporosis at bay. Your provider will assist you in determining the optimal combination of therapies for you and your bone health.

To limit your chance of injury, follow these general safety guidelines:

- Wear your seatbelt at all times.
- Wear the suitable security gear for movements of every sort and sports.
- To avoid tripping yourself or others, keep your house and workspace clutter-free.
- To get to anything around the house, consistently utilize the right apparatuses or hardware. Never put your feet on chairs, tables, or countertops.
- Maintain a healthy diet and workout routine.
- If you have trouble walking or are at risk of falling, use a cane or walker.

CHAPTER 2

Exercise Essentials

Safe and Effective Exercises for Seniors

1. Fast walking

Aerobic exercise is the most common sort of exercise.

Brisk walking is a less intensive sort of aerobic exercise than jogging, but it is still a very useful workout that raises your heart rate and works your muscles. Brisk walking also has a benefit over jogging in that it puts less strain on your joints, so if you have weak knees or ankles, brisk walking is a far better workout option than jogging.

While quick walking may not appear to be an appropriate kind of exercise, you'd be astonished to learn that there are tactics for mastering this sport. Unlike regular walking, brisk walking focuses on improving your gait (how quickly you switch legs) as well as expanding your stride by swinging your hips slightly with each step. Brisk walking also requires proper posture: your back should be straight and your shoulders should be set back for optimal effect.

2. Cycling in a stationary position

Aerobic exercise is the most common sort of exercise.

Stationary bicycles are commonly accessible at most gyms, even those located in community centers. If you prefer to exercise outside, some HDB estates feature fitness corners with stationary bicycles to workout on. Stationary cycling is an excellent kind of cardiovascular exercise, and the greatest part is that it has no stress on your joints, so there is very little risk of damage.

3. Taking a swim

Aerobic exercise is the most common sort of exercise.

Swimming, like cycling, is an excellent type of aerobic exercise since your joints are not overworked because your body weight is supported by the water. Swimming is therefore an excellent form of exercise for people suffering from arthritis and osteoporosis. Furthermore, the added resistance produced by the water provides some benefits for strength training.

Even if you don't know how to swim, going to the pool can be beneficial. Using a swimming board as an aid while paddling certain laps, for example, can help you improve your core and leg muscles. You can also enroll in an aqua aerobics class; you'll be doing a series of water exercises while standing in the pool, so swimming isn't required.

4. squats

Balance is a sort of exercise.

Squats are a quick and easy way to get your daily balance exercise. To begin, you will only need your body weight to perform a squat. You must lower yourself from a standing position into a semi-sitting position for this workout. Squats can be done incorrectly, so keep an eye on your form. Hold your arms out in front of you to maintain your back straight while you squat. Another squat variant is to begin in a chair and gently rise, with your arms extended out parallel to the ground and not grabbing anything for support.

5. Tai Chi

Balance and flexibility exercises

Tai chi is one of the most effective workouts ever devised; it is a low-intensity sport with enormous benefits for one's balance and flexibility. Because tai chi is practiced in groups, it's also a terrific location to meet new exercise buddies. Furthermore, Tai Chi is well-known for being a thoughtful sport that aids in relaxation and focus, making it excellent for mental health as well!

6. Weights for the arms

Strength training is a sort of exercise.

Lifting arm weights not only develops your arms, but also your upper back muscles and shoulders, resulting in better posture and a stronger upper body. Lifting these weights is quite simple: simply begin in a sitting or standing position with the weights held at shoulder level, then lift them all the way up before returning to the original position.

7. Callisthenics

Strength training, balancing exercises

Calisthenics are workouts that use your complete body weight and are an excellent technique to train strength and balance. Push-ups for the arms (on an incline to make it easier), sit-ups (with someone holding your feet in place), and lunges (where you take a big step forward from a standing position to a half-kneeling one while your rear knee hovers just above the ground) are the easiest calisthenics to do.

8. Consistent stretching

Flexibility is a sort of exercise.

Stretching should be done every day because it is an important exercise for keeping your muscles in good shape. Stretch every muscle in your body, including the neck, back, chest, belly, sides, arms, thighs, and calves. Also, work your joints on a daily basis to keep them from stiffening. Your shoulders, hips, knees, and ankles are examples of them.

9. Yoga

Flexibility, balance, and strength training are examples of exercises.

Yoga is a more structured practice of regular stretching exercises that can aid in muscular growth. While you'll be straining your muscles to support your own weight during yoga, this tension won't be too hard on your joints, making yoga ideal for those who have bone or joint problems. Yoga lessons, like Tai Chi, may be a terrific opportunity to meet new people to exercise and bond with, as well as learn mental discipline and attention.

Importance of Balance and Flexibility Training For Seniors

Importance of balance

Why should elders do balance training? As you progress in years, a ton of things change.. Falls can be caused by a variety of factors, including muscle tone, vision, and fundamental limb strength.

According to current research, one out of every five hip fractures in older persons results in death within a year of the incidence. Individuals have a greater mortality rate following a hip fracture due to secondary infection after surgery, pneumonia, and worsening of underlying diseases (the issue that caused the fall in the first place). Of course, there are numerous reasons why seniors should incorporate balance exercise into their routine. Here are a few examples.

Mobility

A decent balance routine combined with a regular exercise routine will assist seniors stay mobile longer than non-exercising contemporaries. The capacity to move without falling and distribute your weight in order to maintain a steady stationary position is referred to as balance. It is similar to anything else in life in that the more you practice, the better it will work.

If you let it, feeling unsteady on your feet can become a vicious cycle. You begin to feel shaky when performing particular activities, and before you know it, you are avoiding those activities and lowering your total mobility. Because you aren't moving as much as you used to, your strength and balance suffer, causing you to be more unstable on your feet.

Several Advantages

Exercise and balance training have numerous advantages for elderly. Here are a few more advantages you can enjoy:

- Exercise and balancing routines help you develop muscle tone, which means better balance and more cushion for your bones if you fall.

- Improved Reaction- If you get somewhat unbalanced, exercise and balance routines give you more time to stop yourself before falling.

- Exercise, particularly resistance training, strengthens bones, resulting in fewer breaks.

- Cognitive Ability- frequent exercise keeps the mind sharp, which means improved processing of your surroundings and the ability to avoid potentially dangerous circumstances.

Overall Wellness

Even if you are not afraid about falling, you should keep in mind that senior fitness and balance routines can assist improve your general health. Stronger muscles and bones, enhanced cardiovascular function, and increased self-confidence are all benefits to your health and well-being.

Things start to change as we get older. Our vision deteriorates, our muscles weaken, and our ability to navigate life becomes difficult. Exercise and balance training are excellent strategies to improve your health and mobility while also boosting your safety at home and in public. There are exercises you can do on your own to improve your balance. You can even go a step further and enroll in a balance-focused fitness class or meet with a Physical Therapist for specialized training. If you live in the Denver area, please contact us to schedule an appointment.

Why Is Senior Flexibility Important?

According to Yogapedia, flexibility is about healthful mobility. It refers to a joint's ability to move over its range of motion. It's also about how soft tissues, such as muscles and tendons, extend and shorten to allow for movement. Staying adaptable has numerous advantages. And, thankfully, there are several simple stretches you can do to enhance your flexibility.

The Benefits of Flexibility

Anyone wondering why flexibility is important for seniors should consider the numerous advantages that acquiring and maintaining flexibility as you age provides. Unique Health & Fitness provides a useful overview:

- Lift the function. Being adaptable makes it easier to execute daily tasks.
- Injury defense. Flexibility improves the risk of injuries such as muscular strains and fractures. It may also contribute to improved balance and a lower risk of falling in seniors.
- Pain reliever. Less chronic pain is related to greater flexibility.
- Improves posture. Stretching can help the spine, neck, and shoulders become more flexible and supple. This reduces the likelihood of obtaining the terrible hunch.
- Improved performance. Flexibility improves muscular performance, thus workouts improve.
- Stress reliever. People who are more flexible are often less anxious because they have less pain, more freedom of movement, and an easier time doing what they want.
- Rejuvenating exercise. People that are adaptable move more effortlessly and confidently. This

gives them a more youthful aspect. Better posture may also result in a more youthful appearance.

Tailoring Exercises to Individual Needs and Abilities

It is critical to build an effective and safe fitness program by tailoring workouts to individual needs and abilities. People's exercise levels, health conditions, ambitions, and preferences differ. Individuals can engage in physical exercise that is appropriate for their own circumstances when using a tailored strategy. Here are some crucial ideas to consider when designing exercises to specific needs and abilities:

1. Evaluation:

- Assess the individual's health status, fitness level, and any pre-existing medical issues thoroughly.
- Age, weight, flexibility, strength, cardiovascular fitness, and any injuries or limits should all be considered.

2. Setting Goals:

- Work with the individual to set clear and attainable fitness goals.
- Weight loss, muscle gain, improved flexibility, increased cardiovascular fitness, or injury recovery are all possible goals.

3. Personal Preferences:

- When it comes to exercising, consider the individual's preferences and dislikes. This raises the likelihood of program adherence.
- Consider your chosen hobbies, workout locations, and time constraints.

4. Development:

- Create a progressive fitness program that begins at a low level and gradually develops in intensity and complexity.
- Reassess the individual's progress on a regular basis and make adjustments as needed.

5. Varieties:

- In order to keep the program interesting and to target different muscle groups, include a variety of activities.
- Include a variety of exercises, including aerobic, strength training, flexibility, and balance activities.

6. Flexibility:

- Prepare to alter exercises based on the individual's response, feedback, or changes in health state.
- Provide workout choices or modifications to fit individual requirements and restrictions.

7. Safety comes first:

- Prioritize safety by avoiding exercises that could endanger the individual's health or aggravate pre-existing illnesses.
- To limit the chance of damage, provide good technique and form teaching.

8. Customized Programming:

- Instead of a one-size-fits-all strategy, create a program that is particularly targeted to the individual.

- Consider your personal preferences for training frequency, duration, and intensity.

9. Education

- Educate the individual on the significance of a well-rounded fitness routine.
- Give information about the advantages of exercise, adequate nutrition, and recovery.

10. Professional Counseling:

Involve fitness specialists, such as personal trainers, physical therapists, or healthcare providers, if possible, to provide expert advice.

Remember that effective exercise programming takes into account the individual's overall well-being, and it's always a good idea to talk with a healthcare practitioner before beginning any new fitness program, especially for people who have pre-existing health concerns.

Chapter 3:

Weight-Bearing Exercises

Gentle Walking Routines

A 9-minute walking exercise for the elderly

Format: Nine minutes of full-body muscular activation and mobility exercises, with each body part focused on separately before combining all motions to practice an optimal walking stride.

Equipment required: Move around freely

Who will benefit from this: Seniors who wish to stretch, mobilize, and stimulate their muscles before going on a stroll.

1. Locate your toes

"I want you to just move your big toe side to side while feeling all of your toes to the ball of your foot as you slightly elevate your heel."

pinky, simply have that psyche to-muscle association," Fichtner proceeds to say.

2. Front-foot rolls

Continue with foot mobilization, but this time from front to back rather than side to side. "Lift the impact point and sort of roll onto the wad of the foot, feeling your toes, then, at that point, lower and afterward substitute," Fichtner said. ""Finally you will essentially start to all around that truly matters, as reasonably run, lifting and moving onto the heaps of the feet."

3. Joint circles in the lower body

Circulate around your joints, beginning with ankle circles on one foot and then the other. Then return to standing on two feet. Circulate your knees one way and then the other with a slight bend in your knees. With your hips, repeat the circle motion. Try to enact your center.

4. Arm swings

This exercise is all about connecting your deep core to movements in your hips and upper body. Stabilize your hips, engage your core, and then begin swinging your arms slightly in front of you, alternating which one is in front.

"With your hips stable first, we will feel this relationship in your thoracic spine over the stomach button," Fichtner said. "Just feel that rotation through the thoracic."

5. Side-to-side hip movements

Get used to moving your hips with balanced and core-connected hips. Rotate them so that each side swerves forward one at a time."It was somewhat side to side, feeling quite free." "I'm not pondering it to an extreme," Fichtner says.

6. Walking practice

Incorporate core-connected mild arm swings into hip side-to-sides to connect the last two exercises.

7. Leg raises

This drill teaches you how to drive from the heel. First, pull your leg up with a bent knee to determine where your natural force comes from. Then you'll concentrate on driving that knee drive from the heel up.

"Lift through the heel," explains Fichtner. "Imagine a mind-to-body link starting from the heel. Consider something raising you from beneath the heel. You don't feel it in your hip flexors or your thighs any longer."

8. Experiment with walking from the sacrum.

"Something last that we will manage is feeling that prolongation," Fichtner said.. You'll do this by locating your sacrum (the bone in your pelvis at the bottom of your spine and just above and between your glutes) and imagining yourself lifting your chest area from the foundation of your spine. This will assist you in pulling the shoulder blades down the back and opening up the chest, allowing your entire body to be erect and lengthened.

"Feel free to take your hands on that sacrum and feel that sacrum," Fichtner proceeds to exhort. "Just stroll around and feel your sacrum. Do you not feel a little taller now? Do you have a longer feeling? How's your posture? Right? Isn't that so much better for the body? "Are you still not rounding forward?"

9. Put everything together

Walk back and forth with a lifted heel, extended spine, and core connection, swaying your hips and swinging your arms.

"We will ponder drooping hips." We'll consider being stretched, feeling long and tall. We'll also consider elevating via the heel."

You're now ready to go.

Low-Impact Aerobics for Bone Density

- Low-impact aerobics can help improve and maintain bone density, especially for people who are at risk of osteoporosis or want to enhance bone health. Here are some low-impact aerobics workouts that may be beneficial:

Walking:

- Walking is a low-impact, weight-bearing activity that is simple to add into your everyday routine.
- To enhance the intensity, aim for brisk walking.

Elliptical Exercise:

- Elliptical machines offer a low-impact cardiovascular workout as well as lower-body exercise.
- The motion is smooth, which reduces joint tension.

Cycling:

- Cycling on a stationary bike or outside is a fantastic low-impact exercise.
- Change the resistance to work your leg muscles and increase bone density.

Swimming:

- Swimming is a non-weight-bearing, joint-friendly workout.
- While it may not have a direct effect on bone density, it does enhance overall fitness and flexibility.

Dancing:

- Low-impact dancing courses or routines can be both fun and beneficial to bone health.
- Avoid high-impact jumps and look for dance genres that stress controlled movements.

Yoga:

- Yoga can help with balance, flexibility, and strength, all of which benefit bone health.

- Concentrate on poses that require you to bear weight on your arms or legs.

Pilates:

- Pilates workouts frequently focus core strength and control.
- Exercises that engage the lower body and incorporate resistance should be included.

Aerobic Classes with Low Impact:

- Many fitness clubs include classes intended exclusively for low-impact aerobics.
- Look for classes that emphasize cardiovascular health without putting too much strain on the joints.

Before beginning any new workout program, it is critical to check with a healthcare practitioner or fitness expert, especially if you have pre-existing health ailments or concerns. They may provide you individualized recommendations based on your specific needs and help ensure that the workouts you choose are safe and effective for increasing bone density. Incorporating strength training exercises and maintaining appropriate calcium and vitamin D intake are also important components of a comprehensive bone health regimen.

Stair Climbing and Step Exercises

Stair climbing and step movements are both good cardio and lower-body workouts. They are convenient and versatile because they can be done practically anywhere there are stairs or step platforms. Here are some advantages and suggestions for stair climbing and step exercises:

Benefits:

Cardiovascular Health:
- Stair climbing raises your heart rate, which benefits your cardiovascular health.
- It improves lung capacity and oxygen absorption.

Lower Body Power:
- Engages important lower-body muscle groups such as the quadriceps, hamstrings, calves, and glutes.
- Tones and strengthens leg muscles.

Calorie Expenditure:
- Provides an efficient method of burning calories, which aids with weight management.

Health of the Joints:

- Stair climbing's low-impact nature is kinder on the joints than high-impact workouts like running.

Convenience:

- It is possible to do it practically anywhere with stairs or a step platform, such as at home, the office, or public places.

Exercises for Stair Climbing:

Stair Climbing in the Old Way:

- Ascend and descend the stairs at a quick rate for a given amount of time.
- Increase the difficulty by taking the stairs two at a time or performing high knees.

Sprints up the stairs:

- Sprint up the stairs for a high-intensity burst of workout.
- For rehabilitation, walk or jog down.

Steps to Take:

Step up the steps sideways to activate different muscular areas.

Lunges:

- Lunges on each step will work the quadriceps and glutes.

Raising Calf:

- Calf raises should be done while standing on the edge of a step.

Step Workouts (With a Step Platform):

Basic Advancement:

- Step one foot up onto the platform, then the other, and then step down.

Step-Ups to the Side:

- Step up to the side, alternately using both legs.

Jumps from a box:

- Jump onto the platform with both feet and land gently.

Kickbacks on Steps:

- For a glute workout, step up with one foot and kick the other leg back.

Intervals of High Intensity:

- Step exercises should be combined with intervals of jumping jacks, burpees, or other high-intensity routines.

Safety Recommendations:

Warm-Up:
- Warm up before beginning strenuous stair or step exercises.

Correct Footwear:
- Wear shoes that are both steady and comfortable.

Posture:
- Maintain proper posture to avoid back and knee discomfort.

Gradual Development:
- Begin with a small number of stairs or a low step height and work your way up.

Before beginning a new fitness plan, contact a healthcare provider, especially if you have any pre-existing health ailments or concerns.

Chapter 4:

Strength Training for Bone Health

Simple Resistance Exercises with Bands or Light weight

7 Easy Resistance Band Exercises For Seniors

1. Pull on the Chest

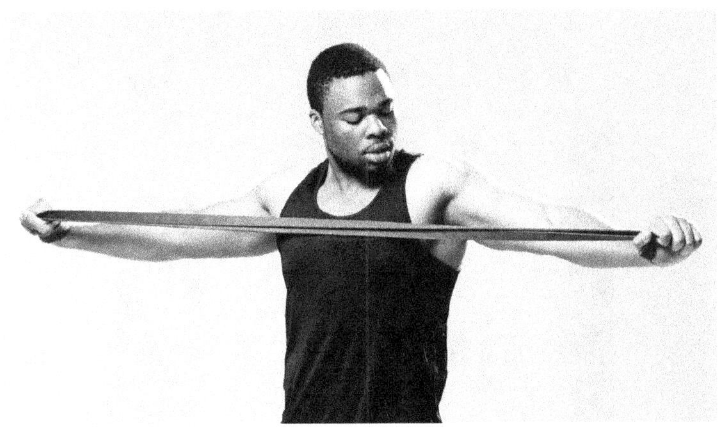

Depending on your preference, you can perform the chest pull in a chair or on your feet. Follow these simple methods to strengthen your upper body once you've decided which one is best for you.

- Grab both ends of your resistance band and place them in front of your chest, elbows bent.
- Take a deep breath in while keeping your back straight and your core engaged.
- Pull the band apart and closer to your chest as you exhale. Fix your arms however much you can.
- Inhale again as you exhale and return to your starting spot.
- Repeat for a total of 10-15 reps.

2. Raise on the Lateral

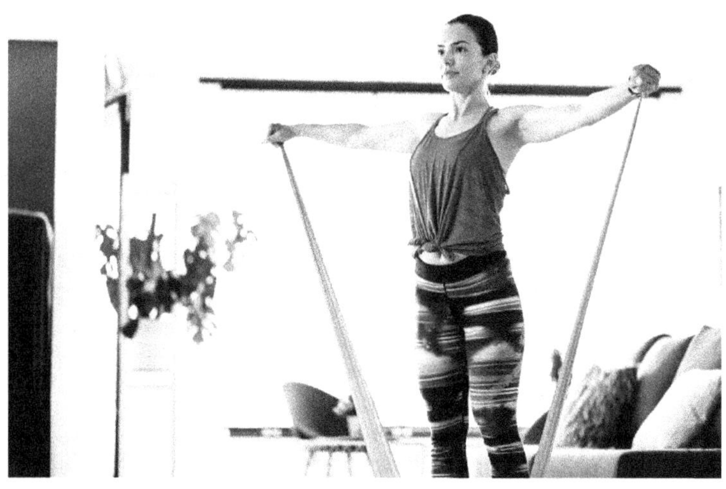

This is a standing workout that will help you improve the muscles around your shoulder blades.

- In the middle of your resistance band, stand shoulder-width apart.
- With your palms facing down and your thumb knuckle pointing forward, grab both ends of your band.
- Raise your arms out to the side to bear level.
- Return to your starting position.
- Repeat for a total of 10-15 reps.

3. Squats

A squat is a complex exercise that engages both the upper and lower bodies.This helps seniors improve the muscular areas they use every day, allowing them to perform daily tasks like getting up and down from a seated position more effortlessly.

- Squats also work your core muscles, which helps your body's general stability and balance.
- Here's how to use your resistance band:
- In the middle of your resistance band, stand shoulder-width apart.
- With your palms facing down and your thumb knuckle pointing forward, grab both ends of your band.

- Pull the band towards your midsection to feel its resistance.
- Slowly bend your knees until you're in a squat position. Maintain a straight back, a flat bottom, and your knees behind your toes.
- Return to your starting point.
- Repeat for a total of 10-15 reps.
- Here's an important thing to remember: You don't have to go all the way to the ground to make this work. Simply get to a point where you feel comfortable and confident in your motions.

4. leg press

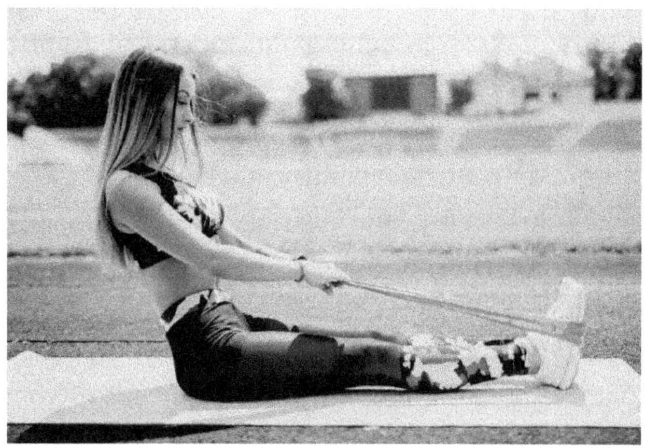

This resistance workout targets your lower body while stretching your leg muscles. You'll require a tough seat for this one.

- Sit in the chair with your back straight and both ends of the resistance band in your hands.
- Place your left foot in the center of the band and extend it out, keeping your right foot firmly planted on the ground.
- Raise your left knee to your chest.
- Straighten it out once more.
- Return your body to the beginning position.
- Switch sides.
- Repeat 10-15 times on each leg.

5. The Calf Press

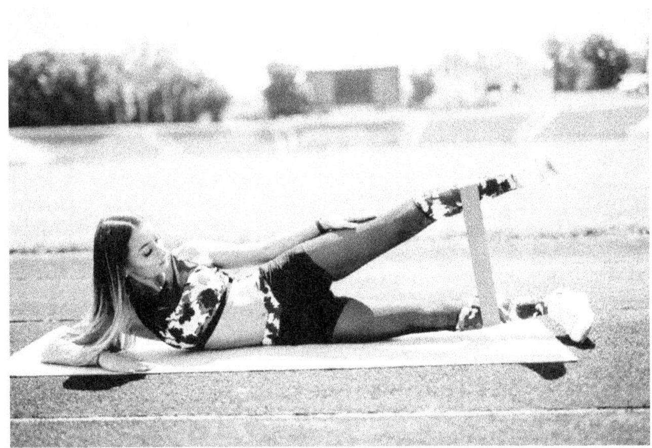

The calf press is another lower-body workout that works your quads, glutes, hamstrings, hips, and (of course) calves. Here's how you can benefit from this workout.

- Sit in the chair with your back straight and both ends of the resistance band in your hands.
- Extend your left foot through the middle of the band.
- Point your toes up to the ceiling once extended.
- Pull your toes back down, pointing them toward the floor.
- Repeat this method 10-15 times back and forth.
- Repeat the process on the other side.

6. Chest Press With a resistance band.

This workout is comparable to a dumbbell chest press, but you don't need a bench to execute it. It can be done either sitting or standing.

- Hold both ends of the resistance band and place the center section behind your back, level with your shoulders.
- Extend your arms so that your hands are directly in front of your chest.
- Return to your starting point.
- Repeat for a total of 10-15 reps.

7. Bent Over Row

Another seated resistance workout is the bent over row. There are also a few variants that might increase the intensity as you become more familiar with the exercises. Here's how to get started:

- Sit in your chair, step on your band, and grab both handles.
- Engage your core, then bend forward until your upper body is parallel to the floor.
- Make sure your hands are facing the ground and your palms are facing backward.
- Place your arms on the ground.
- Pull your hands up to your chest, bringing your shoulder blades closer together. Your elbows will be pointing upwards.
- Return your body to the starting location carefully.
- Repeat for a total of 10-15 reps.
- You can increase the intensity by moving your feet further apart. If it feels too abrasive, you can bring them closer together.

7 Best Senior Dumbbell Exercises

Dumbbell workouts target some of the same muscles as resistance bands, but they are more difficult and carry a larger risk of injury.

Dropping the weights can cause accidents, and poor form can result in muscle tears and other injuries. That is why it is critical to get the motions correct.

Here are a few suggestions to help you reduce your risks:

- Begin with very light weights to get them acclimated to the movements.
- At first, try doing the motions with no weight at all.
- Keep an eye on your form.
- Working with a personal trainer or a spotter will also aid in identifying problem areas.
- As usual, talk with your primary care physician prior to starting.

7 dumbbell workouts for seniors.

Once you are convinced that using dumbbells will not injure your health, you can begin practicing the 7 dumbbell exercises for seniors listed below.

1. Heavy Press

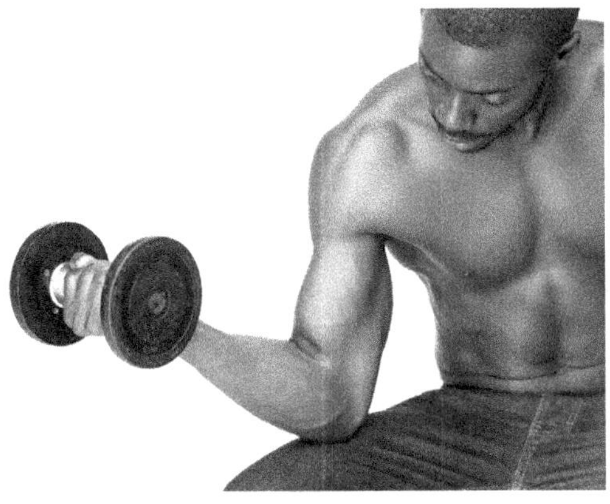

The overhead press can be performed seated or standing. Standing is more difficult since it engages more of your core muscles, but sitting allows you to support your back muscles while working out.

- The remainder of the steps are the same once you've decided how to begin.
- Maintain your posture.
- Grip the dumbbells like handlebars, with your knuckles up and your thumbs on the inside of the dumbbell. This is known as an "overhand grasp."
- Dumbbells should be held at shoulder height.
- Raise your arms over your shoulders and above your head while managing your breathing.
- Maintain this position for one second.
- Return your arms to the beginning position.

- Knowing how many reps to do will depend on your beginning strength, but three sets of 8-12 reps is a good aim.

2. Rows that are bent over

The dumbbell bent over row, commonly known as the dumbbell row, is an excellent exercise for seniors to strengthen their shoulder and back muscles. To finish this movement, follow these means:

- Stand with your knees slightly bent, your feet shoulder-width apart, and your palms facing each other, each holding a dumbbell.
- Bend over 45 degrees at the waist, keeping your back straight.
- Deeply inhale.
- Pull the dumbbells up to your chest as you exhale. Lift the weights no higher than your shoulders and keep your wrists and knees stable while you do so.
- Take another deep breath in and slowly lower the weights to their starting position.
- Repeat the exercise 8-12 times in a session, with a goal of three sets per workout.

3. Raise in the Front

The Front Raise is a basic dumbbell workout that is ideal for beginners to strength training.

- Begin by standing with your hands on your hips and your knees slightly bent. Keep a shoulder-width separation between your feet.
- Using an overhand grip, place the weights between your legs. Maintain your palms facing your body.
- Inhale and contract your abs as you bring your arms straight up with a gentle bend at the elbow.
- When your arms are in a straight line, even with your shoulders, pause.
- Exhale and return the weights to their initial position.
- 8-12 reps in three sets is also a good place to start with this program. If you've never done this before, your weights may range from 5 to 10 pounds, and you can gradually increase as you go.

4. Chest Exercise

The dumbbell chest press involves lying on your back and raising your dumbbells up over your torso. It's typically performed on a training bench, but it can also be performed on the floor or with a Swiss ball if you have one.

This dumbbell workout can assist build important muscle groups in your upper body regardless. This is how it's done:

- Lie on your back and hold your dumbbells horizontally with your knuckles facing your head. Your elbows and shoulders should be aligned, and your arms should be straight.
- Raise your arms above your chest.
- Return your arms to the beginning position.
- Remember to maintain proper form when doing this (and other) moves. Failure to do so can result in damage, so if you're utilizing a bench, be sure your elbows don't slip below your shoulders. Aim for 8-12 reps and three sets of three.

5. Curls on the biceps

Bicep curls are a common dumbbell exercise and one of the best dumbbell exercises you can do. This is most likely the exercise you envision when you think of someone using dumbbells. Here's how to do it correctly:

- Stand erect with your feet flat and your legs shoulder-width apart.
- Hold one dumbbell in each hand, letting your arms naturally fall to your sides. Place your palms outward.
- Bend your elbows and lift the weight to your chest. Your arms should be solid and your shoulders should be relaxed.
- Return the weights to their initial position slowly.
- Rep 8-12 times more in three sets.

6. Squat with Dumbbells

The dumbbell squat is a complex exercise, which means that it works both the upper and lower body. This helps seniors improve the muscular areas they use every day, allowing them to perform daily tasks like getting up and down from a seated position more effortlessly.

Furthermore, the dumbbell squat targets your core muscles, allowing you to improve your body's overall stability and balance.

This is how it's done:

- Hold the end of one dumbbell in the center of your chest with both hands.
- Make your legs broader than your hips. Maintain a flat foot with your toes pointed forward or slightly turned out.
- Tighten your core, then bend your knees and hips into a squatting stance.
- When your legs are parallel to the floor, come to a halt. (At first, you might not make it that far. That's all right. Simply go as low as you can while keeping proper form.)
- Return your body to an upright position.

Because squats work your entire body, you may discover that you can use more weight than with other exercises. However, don't push yourself too hard because you don't want to injure yourself, and remember that you don't have to go all the way down to the ground. You should choose a position that allows you to feel secure and confident, just like with the resistance bands.

7. Triceps Extension While Lying

This is a triceps isolation workout that focuses on the lower arm. This exercise, like the chest press, works best with a bench.

- Lie on a bench with your hands extended out and over your chest, holding a dumbbell in each.
- Bend your elbows so that the weights fall below your shoulders.
- Maintain your upper arms' stability.
- For a brief moment, pause at the bottom.
- Return the weights to their starting position.
- As you begin, repeat with 8-12 reps and 2 sets.

How Exercise Aids Seniors in Avoiding Falls

A regular fitness routine can go a long way toward preventing falls in seniors. As your body strengthens, so do your flexibility, balance, and mobility.

Incorporating dumbbell movements or resistance training into your workout program will provide your body with the support it requires to stay upright.

Always maintain appropriate form, rest when necessary, and quit training if you feel your body can't do it.

Consult your doctor about the best exercises for you, especially if you have a medical condition. Nothing we've said here should be construed as professional medical advice. You ought to in any case talk with an expert.

When you have the all-ahead, you can go out and buy some dumbbells and a resistance band to start reaping the benefits of these exercises.

Bodyweight Exercises for Strength and Stability

Seniors must prioritize workouts that enhance strength, flexibility, balance, and total functional fitness while taking into account any current health issues or limits. Prior to starting another wellness plan, consistently talk with a medical care professional. Here are some bodyweight exercises that are appropriate for seniors:

Leg Lifts While Sitting:

Quadriceps and hip flexors are the muscles targeted.

- Sit in a chair and raise one leg straight out in front of you, then lower it back down.

Chair Squats:

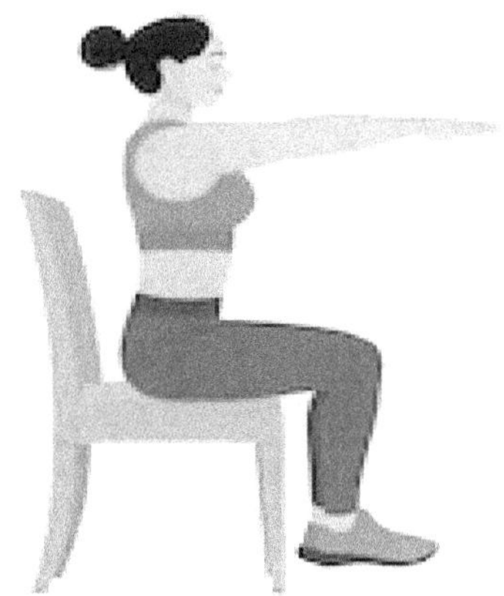

Support with a chair

Quadriceps, hamstrings, and glutes are the muscles targeted.

- Use a firm chair for support, then stand up and sit back down with proper form.

Wall Push-Ups:

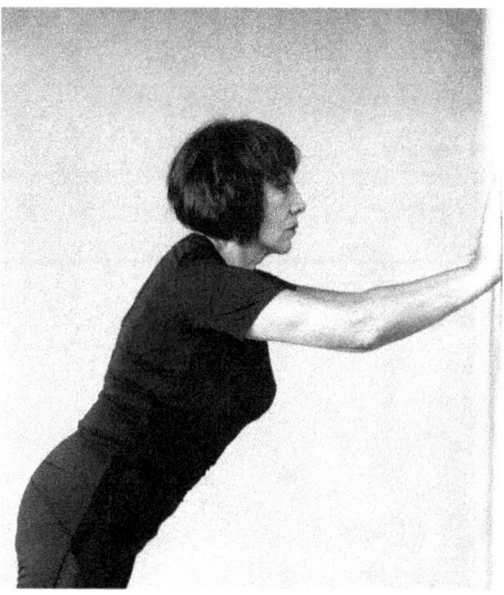

Chest, shoulders, and triceps are the muscles targeted.

- Perform push-ups against a wall while standing at arm's length from it.

Calves are the primary target of standing calf raises.

- Hold on to a solid surface and rise onto your toes before lowering your heels.
- Targets for seated marching include core muscles and hip flexors.
- Sit on the edge of a chair and raise your knees one at a time, as if marching.

Quadriceps are the muscles targeted by leg extensions.

- Sit on a chair and elevate one leg straight out in front of you, one at a time.

Side Leg Raises:

Outer thighs and hip abductors are targeted.

- Lift one leg out to the side and lower it back down behind a sturdy chair.

Cardiovascular fitness and leg muscles are targeted via toe taps.

- Sit in a chair and swiftly tap your toes on the floor.

Arm Circles:

Shoulders and arms are the targets.

- Sit or stand with your arms at your sides, doing circular motions with your arms.

Neck Stretches:

To enhance neck flexibility, gently tilt your head from side to side, forward and backward.

Torso Twists While Sitting:

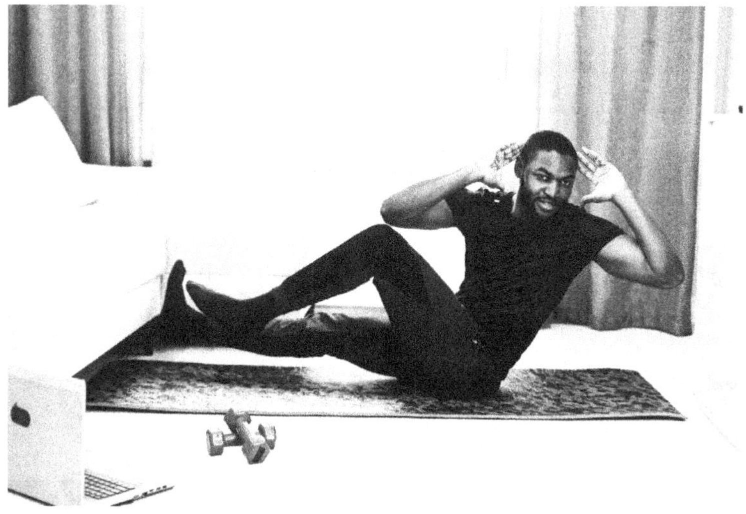

- Sit on a chair with your feet flat on the ground and rotate your torso from side to side.
- Walking in a straight line with the heel of one foot directly in front of the toes of the other improves balance.
- Walking at a reasonable speed, even if only around the house or in the yard, can be an excellent method to preserve cardiovascular health.

Deep Breathing Exercises:

- Concentrate on taking deep, regulated breaths to increase lung capacity and relaxation.

Senior Yoga or Tai Chi:

These low-impact activities combine gentle movements, stretching, and breathing techniques to promote balance and flexibility.

- Warm up first, then listen to your body and alter workouts as needed. The goal is to maintain and develop overall mobility, strength, and balance while taking individual talents and medical concerns into account.

Tips for Gradual Progression

Gradual exercise development is essential for seniors to maintain and enhance their health and fitness while limiting the chance of injury. Here are some suggestions geared specifically for seniors:

Consultation with a Medical Professional:

- Consult your healthcare practitioner before beginning any fitness program to ensure it is safe for your specific health condition.

Begin with low-intensity exercises:

- Begin with low-influence exercises like strolling, swimming, or cycling.
- As your fitness increases, gradually increase the duration and intensity.

Warm-Up and Cool-Down:

- Incorporate a good warm-up and cool-down into your exercise program to prepare your muscles and joints and avoid injury.

Concentrate on adaptability:

- Stretching activities should be used to increase flexibility and range of motion.
- Yoga and tai chi are great exercises for improving balance and flexibility.

Light Weight Strength Training:

- Include strength training routines that use light weights or resistance bands.

- To progressively gain strength, focus on repeated repetitions with decreased resistance.

Balance Exercises:

- Include balance exercises in your routine to lower your chance of falling.
- Simple tasks such as standing on one leg or walking heel-to-toe can help improve balance.

Pay Attention to Your Body:

- Pay attention to how your body reacts to exercise.
- Adjust the intensity or type of exercise if you encounter pain or discomfort.

Stay Hydrated:

Staying hydrated is critical, especially for seniors.

- Remain hydrated by drinking water previously, during, and after work out.

Intensity and Consistency:

- Seniors require consistency. Regular, moderate exercise is more beneficial than intensive workouts on occasion.

- Go for the gold 150 minutes out of every seven day stretch of moderate-power work out.

Use Correct Form:

- Maintain appropriate form during activities to avoid strain or injury.
- Consider working with a fitness professional for technique advice.

Modify as Needed:

- Don't be afraid to change routines to accommodate your fitness level and any physical restrictions.
- For those who have mobility limitations, chair workouts or sitting modifications can be beneficial.

Track Progress:

- Maintain a record of your exercise program and track your development over time.
- Adjust your plan in response to any improvements or changes in your health.

Include Aerobic Workout:

- Improve your cardiovascular health by engaging in aerobic activities such as brisk walking, swimming, or dancing.
- Strive for a mix of aerobic and strength training workouts.

Socialize and Have Fun:

- Exercising with others can make it more fun.
- To keep motivated, consider taking group classes or finding an exercise buddy.

Take your time:

- Understand that progress may take time, and that you must be patient with yourself.
- Celebrate tiny victories and landmarks along the path.

Seniors can accept progressive growth in their exercise routines by following these guidelines, improving overall well-being and keeping a healthy lifestyle. Always put safety first, pay attention to your body, and reap the benefits of regular physical activity.

CHAPTER 5.

Balance and Stability

Balance Exercises to Reduce Fall Risk

As we age, falls can have significant repercussions. According to the Centers for Disease Control and Prevention, more than 25% of persons 65 and over fall each year, and 3 million are treated in emergency departments for fall injuries.

Fall Risks

In most cases, the risk of falling in older persons is connected to a mix of factors, including:

- Problems with balance and/or walking. Vision alterations, vestibular issues, and changes in foot sensation can all have an impact on balance.
- The usage of several drugs. According to research, taking five or more medications increases the risk of falling.
- Home dangers (such as poor illumination and trip hazards)

- Positional hypotension (such as orthostatic hypotension, which occurs when blood pressure lowers upon standing.
- Problems with the feet and footwear

Falls occur frequently in the bathroom when sitting or standing from the toilet or shower, or at night in a dark bedroom when waking up fast and tripping on the way to the bathroom.

Falls Prevention Exercises

While it is difficult to thoroughly abstain from falling, exercises that focus on equilibrium and strength preparing assist with reducing the possibility of falling. "I treat elderly adults who have been injured in falls, as well as other patients who feel unsteady while walking or standing and are afraid of falling,"Activities such as squatting, standing up from a chair, and walking may be difficult or unsteady for older persons, increasing their risk of falling. The following exercises are designed for people who have a low risk of falling and can stand on their own without assistance. Before beginning new workouts, always consult with your doctor or physical therapist, especially if you have poor balance.

Sit-to-Stand Workout

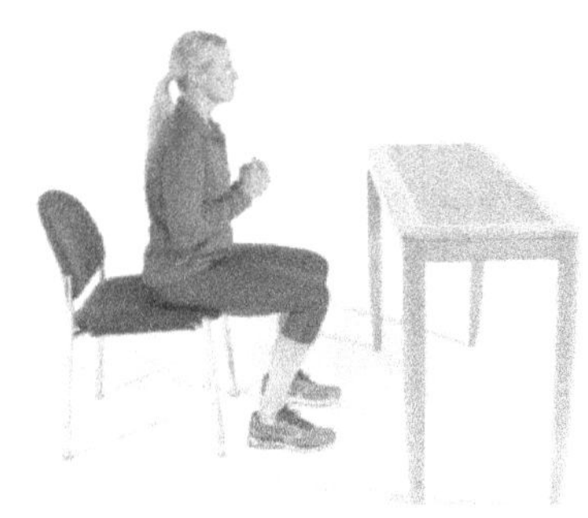

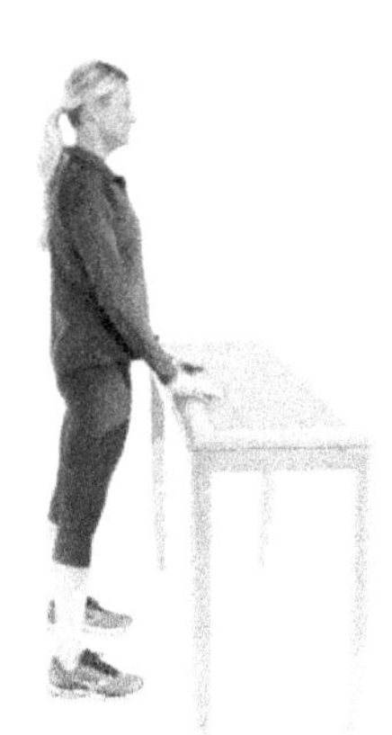

The sit-to-stand exercise increases leg strength while also improving body mechanics and balance, all of which are helpful in preventing falls.

1. Begin by sitting in a sturdy chair that is of regular height and does not slip or roll. Your feet should be flat on the ground and you should be able to sit comfortably. Keep a firm support surface in front of you, such as a countertop, so you can grab it for assistance if you begin to feel unstable while standing. Move forward so your buttocks are at the front of the seat.

2. Shift your entire weight forward by leaning your chest forward over your toes. Squeeze your gluteal muscles and steadily raise yourself to a standing position.

3. Return to the starting position slowly and repeat 10 times.

4. If necessary, place your hands on the chair's armrests or seat and push through your hands to assist in standing and sitting. The idea is to avoid using your hands at all costs.

Do ten repetitions twice a day. Hold hand weights to provide resistance for a more advanced variant.

If you experience pain in your knees, back, or hips, stop and consult your doctor or physical therapist.

Balance Training

If your balance is shaky, try this set of exercises. Make sure someone is nearby in case you lose your balance.

To begin, stand in a corner or have a kitchen counter in front of you to grasp for if you begin to lose your balance.

1. Feet apart:

- Stand with your feet shoulder-width apart, eyes wide, and hold for 10 seconds, gradually increasing to 30 seconds.
- If you find yourself wobbling or grabbing for the wall or counter frequently, just keep practicing until you can do it with little swaying or support. Move on to the next exercise once you can hold this position solidly for 30 seconds.

2. Feet together:

- Stand with your feet together, eyes open, and hold for 10 seconds, gradually increasing to 30 seconds.

- Move on to the next one once you can do this one for 30 seconds with minimal wobbling or support.

3. One foot:

- Stand on one foot, eyes open, and hold for 10 seconds, gradually increasing to 30 seconds. Change to the other foot.

4. Closed eyes:

- If you can complete the first three exercises safely and with minimal assistance, try each one with your eyes closed. Hold for 10 seconds, gradually increasing to 30 seconds.

The goal for each exercise is to hold the position for 10 seconds and gradually proceed to 30 seconds, five repetitions (five per leg on the one-foot exercise), two times per day.

Additional Fall Prevention Falls

- Remember to consult your doctor or physical therapist about fall prevention.
- Discuss drugs and modifications to your workout program with your doctor.
- If you fall, notify your doctor.
- Ask a friend or family member to assist you in inspecting your home for trip risks.

"Keep in mind," I goes on to say, "it is always best to have company at home with you while exercising for safety and supervision and in case you need help."

Incorporating Tai Chi and Yoga for Improved Stability

Including Tai Chi and Yoga in your regimen will help you improve your stability, balance, flexibility, and overall well-being. Both traditions have ancient origins and are concerned with the mind-body link. Here's how you can enhance your stability by combining Tai Chi and

Yoga:

1. Begin with thoughtful Breathing:

Begin each session with some deep, thoughtful breathing. This assists in centering your mind and relaxing your body in preparation for the workouts ahead.

2. Begin with a light warm-up that includes yoga poses that emphasize balance and flexibility, such as Tree Pose, Warrior Pose, and Sun Salutations. This assists with heating up your muscles and joints.

3. Include Tai Chi for Balance:

Tai Chi focuses on gentle, flowing movements that engage the entire body. Slow transitions between postures improve your stability and aid in the development of a fine sense of balance. Consider including Tai Chi motions such as "Grasp the Sparrow's Tail" or "Parting the Wild Horse's Mane."

4. Incorporate Yoga and Tai Chi Poses:

Incorporate Tai Chi exercises into your yoga program. Incorporate Tai Chi-inspired leg swings or arm movements, for example, into your standing yoga positions. This combination promotes a smooth transition between the two practices.

5. encourage Core Strength:

Tai Chi and Yoga both encourage core activation. Yoga poses like Boat Pose and Tai Chi moves like "Punching with Angry Eyes" strengthen your core muscles and promote stability.

6. Mindful Transitions:

Pay attention to how you change stances. This attention is essential to both Tai Chi and Yoga. Move purposefully and mindfully, activating the muscles required for stability.

7. Use Props:

Using props such as yoga blocks or a firm chair will help you improve your stability. Use them to change poses or to assist as needed.

8. Yoga Stretches to Cool Down:

Finish your workout with yoga stretches that focus on flexibility and relaxation. Poses such as Child's Pose, Cobra, and Downward-Facing Dog can assist relieve stress.

9. Conclude with Meditation:

Finish your practice with a brief meditation. Both Tai Chi and Yoga emphasize mental clarity and attention.

Meditation can help you improve your concentration and overall well-being.

10. Practice on a regular basis to see improvements. These techniques' advantages compound over time, improving your stability, balance, and general physical and mental health.

11. Adapt to Your Situation:

Change the poses and motions to suit your degree of comfort and physical condition. Pay attention to your body and progress slowly as you get more comfortable with the exercises.

Before beginning a new workout plan, talk with a healthcare practitioner or fitness expert, especially if you have any existing health concerns or conditions. Consider taking a class or working with a trained instructor to ensure that you're doing the moves correctly and securely.

Functional Movements for Everyday Activities

Functional movements are very important for seniors because they help them stay independent and improve their quality of life generally. These moves are good for seniors and can help them:

1. Squatting:

- This moves like getting up from a chair, going to the bathroom, or picking up things off the ground.
- Squats with your own body weight or chair squats.
- Lunging is like walking, going up and down stairs, or reaching for things.
- Do lunges in front of you, behind you, or to the side.

3. Balancing:

- This is the same thing as keeping your balance while walking or standing.
- Stand on one leg, walk from heel to toe, or balance on one foot.

4. Walking:

Looks like:

Normal walking.

As an exercise, you can go for brisk walks, walks on different types of terrain, or short walks.

5. Pushing and Pulling:

Mimics: Opening doors, pushing a shopping cart, or pulling a heavy item.

Exercise: Standing chest press, seated row, or resistance band movements.

6. Gait Training:

Mimics:Improving the pattern of walking.

Exercise:

Walking with exaggerated steps, high knees, or toe walking.

7. Reaching and Stretching:

Mimics: Reaching for things on shelves or putting on/taking off clothes.

Exercise: Overhead reaches, side stretches, or reaching for toes.

8. Core Strengthening:

Mimics: Maintaining stability during different activities.

Exercise: Seated leg lifts, seated knee extensions, or sitting bicycle crunches.

9. Twisting Movements: Mimics: Turning to look behind or reaching for things to the side.

Exercise: Seated or standing body twists.

10. Functional Step-Ups:

Mimics: Climbing stairs or stepping up onto a barrier.

Exercise: Step-ups on a sturdy platform.

11. Gentle Arm Exercises:

Mimics: Reaching, lifting, and carrying lightweight items.

Exercise: Arm circles, bicep curls with light weights, or resistance band movements.

12. Gentle Neck Movements:

Mimics: Turning the head to look around or up and down.

Exercise: Neck stretches and twists.

13. Joint Flexibility Exercises:

Mimics: Maintaining joint mobility for daily tasks.

Exercise: Range of motion movements for the wrists, ankles, shoulders, and hips.

14. Functional Sit-to-Stand:

Mimics: Getting in and out of a car or standing from a low seat.

Exercise: Sit-to-stand movements, gradually raising the height of the chair.

15. Tai Chi Movements:

Mimics: Fluid and controlled movements for general balance and coordination.

Exercise: Tai Chi routines focusing on gentle, flowing movements.

16. Water Aerobics:

Mimics: Provides resistance for different movements.

Exercise: Water aerobics can be gentler on joints while offering a full-body workout.

Always prioritize safety and speak with a healthcare professional or fitness expert before starting a new exercise routine. Exercises should be adapted to individual abilities and grow gradually. Additionally, consider group classes or activities for social involvement and motivation.

Chapter 6:

Flexibility and Range of Motion

Gentle Stretching for Improved Flexibility

Stretching Exercises for Seniors

1. Standing Quadriceps Stretch

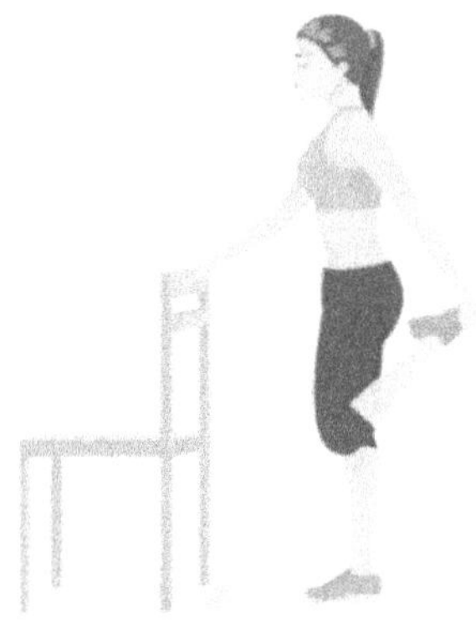

The first exercise on our list is the standing thigh stretch. As a crucial exercise for mobility and flexibility, the standing quadriceps stretch is an excellent stretching exercise for adults.

As the largest extremities, the legs may require multiple stretches for the full benefits these stretches give. This exercise focuses on the quadriceps muscle, found on the top half of your upper leg.

To start:

- Make sure you loosen up before stretching by doing some light walking around.
- Grab a chair or the back of a couch for support, as you will be standing on one leg for this exercise. The stronger the support, the better.
- Clutch the seat with your left hand. Bend your right knee, and, using your right hand, grab your leg by the ankle and slowly pull your foot towards your bottom.
- Hold this pose for 10 to 30 seconds, let your leg back down and repeat with your left leg.
- For folks that have problems when standing up, you can try the seated ankle stretch, which also serves as a great stretch for your quadriceps.

2. Seated Knee to Chest

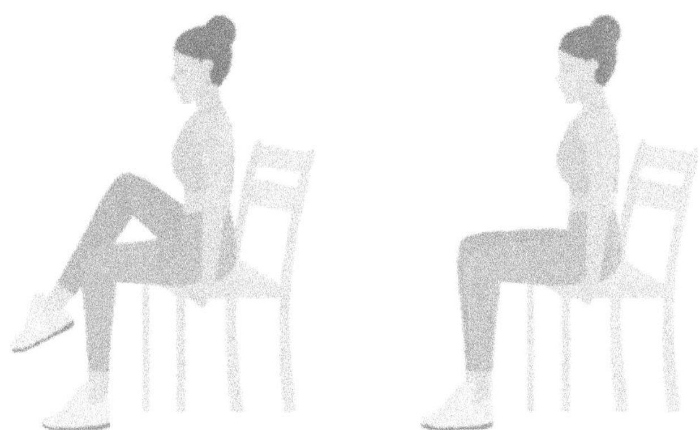

This lower body stretch is a necessary exercise for adults as it impacts more than just your legs. The knee to chest stretching exercise improves movement in your hips and knees by stretching the joints, while also improving the flexibility of your lower back. A nice extra bonus about this stretch is that you don't need to stand!

Here's how to get started:

- Like the last exercise, stretch up a bit by doing some light walking to warm up your legs.
- Sit comfortably in your chair, and while sitting, grasp your right knee and slowly pull it towards your chest.

- Once you feel the stretching sensation, hold this pose for 10 to 30 seconds.
- Gently guide your leg back down to the floor and repeat this movement with your other leg.

[iorablogcta]

3. Hamstring Stretch

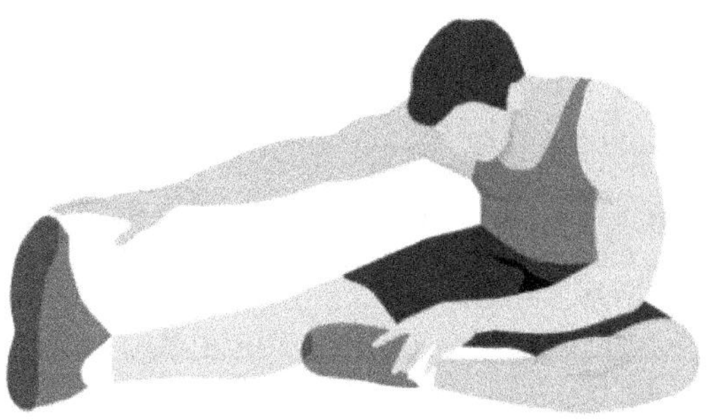

Now that we've covered your quadriceps and your hips, now is the ideal time to show your hamstrings a tad of adoration.

This stretching exercise targets your lower back and your legs, a crucial component for keeping flexibility in seniors. This stretch will decrease stiffness and keep your legs and back mobile and open.

To start the stretch:

- Select a hard surface to sit on.
- Next, stretch one of your legs out on the surface.
- Gradually incline forward, inhale and go after your thigh, knee or lower leg.(Be careful with this stretch as you do not want to hyperextend your leg). Next, hold this pose for 10 to 30 seconds and gently lay your leg back down and repeat with the other side of your body.

4. Soleus Stretch

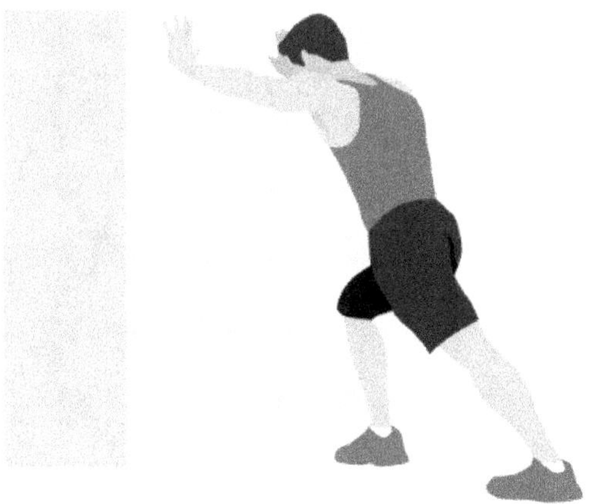

This simple stretch is great for another big muscle group in your legs: the calf muscle. The soleus stretch targets your calves and lower body flexibility by improving the deep calf muscle and the general functionality of your legs.

To start this stretching exercise:

- Stand up and face a wall.
- Place your right foot in front of your left and place both hands on the wall in front of you for support. Once you feel relaxed, begin to slowly bend your knees until you begin to feel a stretch in your lower leg. Hold this pose for 10 to 30 seconds. After you feel good and stretched, slowly stand up, swap the places of your left and right feet and repeat the exercise again.

5. Overhead Side Stretch

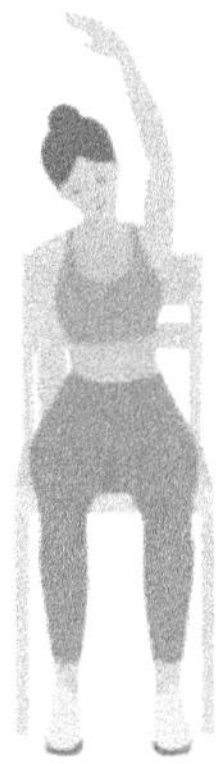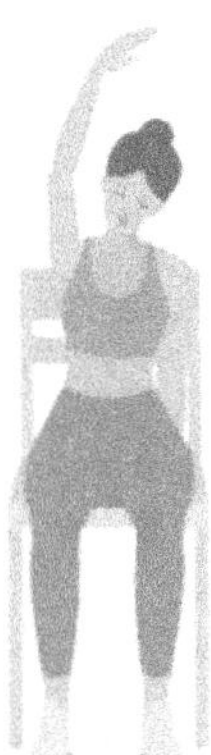

Fifth on our list of workouts, we will start with the upper body! The overhead side stretch, or standing side stretch, is a great and easy way to loosen up your belly, back and shoulders.

To start:

- Stand with your feet shoulder-width apart and raise your arms over your head, linking your fingers if you'd like.
- Keeping your body long, slowly lean to the left. Hold this pose for 10 to 30 seconds, return to the center; Repeat the same stretch on the right side. *Another great feature of this exercise is that you can do it while sitting down.

- For older folks with mobility or health complications, this exercise can be performed in a similar way:
- Sit in a tall chair and keep your hips, knees and toes looking forward.
- Lift your arms above your head and repeat the steps above. (If you find this too tough, place your arms on your hips, or down to your side).
- Gently lean to either side for 10 to 30 seconds.

6. Shoulder Stretch

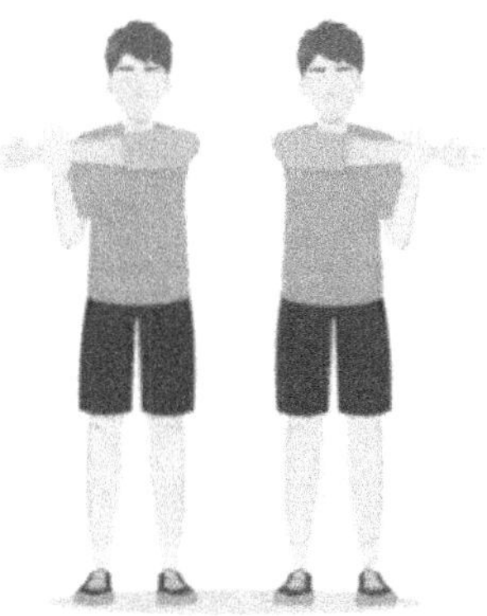

For our next stretch, we'll stay with the upper body and work on shoulders. With this simple shoulder stretch, you can loosen up your shoulder joint, which can be used to alleviate muscle pain and avoid deterioration.

Here's how you should start:

- Stand, or sit straight up, as tall as possible.
- Grab one of your arms with your opposite hand and slowly, gently pull your arm across your chest until you start to feel a stretch in your shoulder. (While you stretch, make sure that you keep your arm below shoulder height).
- Hold this pose for 10 to 30 seconds and then repeat with your other arm.

Similar as the activity before this, you can play out this stretch while standing or sitting, whichever you like to benefit from your extended workout.

7. Tricep Stretch

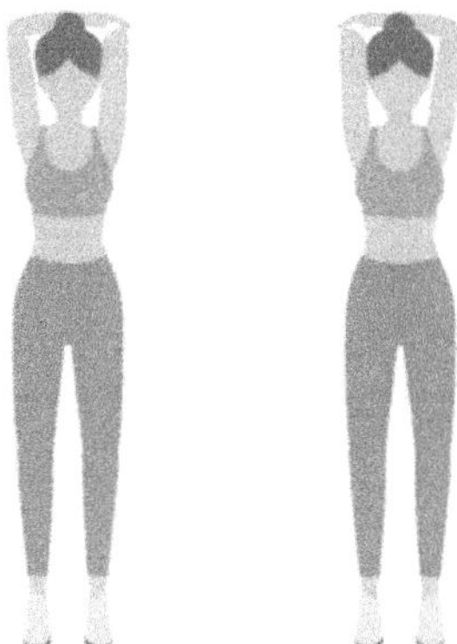

The tricep stretch is the next on our list, but the last for our upper body. The tricep stretch, while designed to extend your arms, is also an excellent approach to enhance shoulder mobility.

The tricep stretch, like the rest of our upper body exercises, can be done standing or sitting. Simply sit tall and utilize a chair to keep your back straight!

To start

- Stand or sit tall with your feet hip-width separated.

- Raise both arms above your head, bending your right arm to place it behind your head.
- Place your left hand on your right elbow and gradually draw it down towards your back until you feel stretching in your upper arm.
- Hold for 10 to 30 seconds, then return your arms to their original position and repeat the stretch with your left arm.

8. Advanced Lunge in a Chair

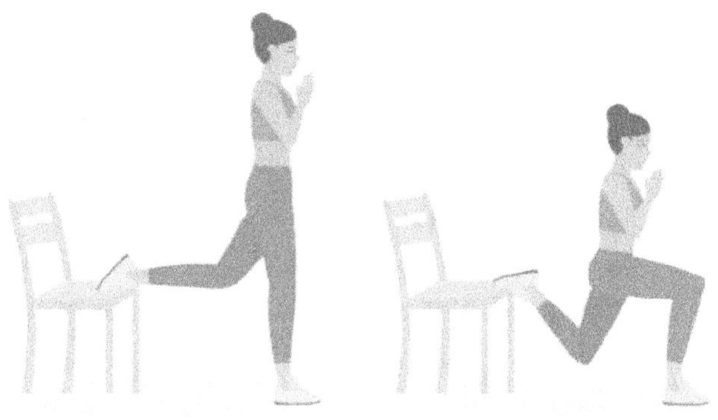

So far, we've covered a variety of muscle groups and talked extensively about your upper and lower bodies, but what about the area in between? This stretching exercise is ideal for seniors who want to preserve their mobility and muscle strength. This activity, however, is not required because it can be challenging. Listen to your body and only do this workout if you are capable.

To begin:

- Place two strong chairs about three feet apart, facing the same direction.
- Next, step a few steps in front of the chair behind you and rest your shin on the seat. Your knee should extend slightly over the front border of the chair, with your foot dangling over the back.
- Then, slightly bend your front leg while moving your hips forward and down. Hold this position for 10 to 30 seconds before repeating on the opposing side.

9. Advanced Standing Hip Flexor

The standing hip flexor stretch is the last but not least on our list of stretches for seniors. This stretch, one of many hip flexor stretches for seniors, is an excellent approach to relieve hip tightness or pain. It should be mentioned, however, that this is a demanding workout that may be better suited for more advanced individuals. Here's how **to go about it:**

- First, take a strong chair and stand with your feet facing the back of the chair, leaving enough space between yourself and the chair to pull your leg up.

- Then, while hanging on to the chair with both hands, lift your opposing leg towards your chest with your knee bent, putting your knee as near to your chest as possible.
- Hold this position for 10 to 15 seconds before repeating with the opposite leg.

What Should You Do After Stretching?

After you've finished your stretching exercises, it's time to think about other ways to improve your health. Proper hydration, exercise, and diet, along with stretching activities, all contribute to seniors' general health.

Yoga and Pilates for Joint Mobility

Yoga and Pilates are both great exercises for improving joint mobility, flexibility, and overall joint health. You can improve joint range of motion and reduce stiffness by incorporating specific poses and exercises. Here's how to utilize Yoga and Pilates to improve joint mobility:

Cat-Cow Stretch (Chakravakasana) for Joint Mobility:

- It focuses on the spine, shoulders, and hips.
- Encourages spine flexibility and mobility.
- Adho Mukha Svanasana (Downward-Facing Dog): Stretches the shoulders, hamstrings, and calves.
- Increases shoulder and ankle mobility.

Warrior Poses (Virabhadrasana I, II, III): These poses work the hips, knees, and ankles.

- Improves lower-body flexibility and strength.
- Stretches the spine, hamstrings, and shoulders with seated forward bend (Paschimottanasana).
- Improves hip and lower back flexibility.

Pigeon Pose (Eka Pada Rajakapotasana):

- This pose focuses on the hips and thighs.
- Improves hip mobility and flexibility.

Malasana (Garland Pose):

- This pose focuses on the ankles, knees, and hips.
- It aids in the opening of the hip joints.

Bridge Pose (Setu Bandhasana):

- This posture strengthens the spine, hips, and chest.
- It increases spinal flexibility and leg strength.
- Stretches the hamstrings and hips in Supine Hand-to-Big-Toe Pose (Supta Padangusthasana).
- Improves leg and hip joint flexibility.

Pilates Exercises for Joint Mobility:

- The Saw focuses on the spine, shoulders, and hips.
- Improves spine rotation and flexibility.

Leg Circles:

- This exercise focuses on hip mobility.
- Improves hip joint flexibility and strength.

The Hundred:

- This exercise works the shoulders, arms, and core.
- Increases shoulder joint mobility.

Swan Dive:

- This exercise focuses on the spine and shoulders.
- Increases spine flexibility and expands the chest.
- The Side Leg Lift Series targets the hips and thighs.
- Increases the mobility and strength of the hip joint.

Scissors:

- This exercise works the hip flexors and hamstrings.
- Stretches the hamstrings and improves hip flexibility.

Corkscrew:

- This exercise focuses on spine rotation.
- Aids in the improvement of spine mobility.

- Rolling Like a Ball: This exercise targets the spine and engages the core.
- This exercise improves spinal flexibility and coordination.

Yoga and Pilates Joint Mobility Tips:

aware Movement:

- To avoid tension, focus on controlled and aware motions.

Warm-up:

- To prepare joints for activity, begin each session with a mild warm-up.

good Alignment:

- Pay attention to good alignment in postures to avoid extra joint tension.

Breath Awareness:

- Align your breath with your activity to improve relaxation and joint flexibility.

Modify as Needed:

- Adjust poses and exercises to accommodate individual abilities and any existing joint concerns.
- Consistency is essential for improving joint mobility over time.

Consult a healthcare physician or fitness expert before beginning any new exercise plan, especially if you have joint difficulties or health issues. They may advise you on suitable adaptations and ensure that the exercises you choose are safe and effective for your individual condition.

Including Stretching in Your Daily Routine

Stretching as part of your daily regimen can improve flexibility, reduce muscle tension, and promote general well-being. Here's how to incorporate stretching into your daily routine:

1. Morning Stretch Routine:

- Begin your day by gently stretching your muscles and increasing blood flow.
- Neck stretches, shoulder rolls, spinal twists, and hamstring stretches should be prioritized.
- Include active stretches to help your body ready for the day.

2. Desk Stretches (For Office Workers):

- If you work at a desk, take short breaks every hour to stand up and stretch.
- Stretch your neck, shoulders, wrists, and lower back while seated.
- Include standing exercises like calf lifts and hip flexor stretches.

3. Lunchtime Stretch Break:

- Take advantage of your lunch break to perform a brief stretching routine.
- Concentrate on key muscular groups such as the neck, shoulders, back, and legs.
- Include some deep breathing exercises to help you relax.

4. Afternoon Pick-Me-Up Stretch:

- Avoid afternoon tiredness by stretching for a few minutes.
- Include chest, wrist, and hip flexor stretches.
- Gentle backbends should be used to stretch your spine.

5. Post-Work Stretching Session:

- Set aside time after work for a longer stretching exercise.
- All main muscular groups, including the legs, back, shoulders, and hips, should be targeted.
- In order to increase flexibility and strength, incorporate yoga positions or Pilates workouts.

6. Evening Stretch Routine:

- Relax in the evening by performing soothing stretches to relieve tension.
- Stretches that promote relaxation, such as moderate forward bends and hip openers, should be prioritized.
- For a relaxing impact, incorporate deep breathing or meditation.

7. Stretching While Watching TV:

- Use your TV time to stretch.

- During your favorite shows, do seated or laying stretches for your legs, hips, and back.

8. Stretching Before Bed:

- To relax your body, incorporate mild stretches into your evening regimen.
- Stretches that promote better sleep, such as hamstring stretches and moderate twists, should be prioritized.
- For a restful night, combine stretching with deep breathing or meditation.

9. Weekend Flexibility Session:

- Set aside more time on weekends for an in-depth flexibility session.
- To mix things up, try longer yoga exercises or a stretching class.
- For a holistic approach, concentrate on both static and dynamic stretches.

10. Pay Attention to Your Body:

- Pay attention to how your body feels and alter your regimen as needed.
- If you are tight or sore, prioritize mild stretching over strenuous exercise.

11. Consistency is Key:

- Make stretching a daily practice to reap long-term benefits.
- Even brief, consistent exercises can result in increased flexibility and decreased stiffness.
- 12. Incorporate Stretching into Other Activities: Incorporate stretching into other activities like walking or jogging.
- Stretch dynamically before exercising and statically afterwards.

13. Stay Hydrated:

- Stay hydrated because dehydration can add to muscle stiffness.

14. Use Props and Tools:

- To deepen stretches, use props such as yoga blocks or resistance bands.
- For myofascial release, consider utilizing a foam roller.

Always stretch gradually and without bouncing, and always listen to your body. Before beginning a new stretching regimen, talk with a healthcare practitioner or fitness expert if you have any health concerns or current issues.

Chapter 7:

Lifestyle and Nutrition

Importance of Calcium and Vitamin D

For adults, calcium and vitamin D are even more important because their bones become less dense with age, they may fall more often, and their bodies may not absorb nutrients as well. This is why calcium and vitamin D are especially important for older people:

Calcium:

Good for bones and preventing osteoporosis:

Osteoporosis makes bones weak and fragile, and older people are more likely to get it. Getting enough calcium helps keep bones strong and lowers the risk of breaking them.

Function of Muscles:

 Calcium is needed for muscles to work right, and adults need it to keep their muscles strong and not fall.

Joint Health:

Calcium is good for joint health and helps you move around and be flexible.

Blood Pressure Control:

Calcium may help seniors enjoy better heart health by helping to keep their blood pressure in check.

Dental Problems:

Getting enough calcium is important for keeping your teeth healthy and avoiding dental problems that can hurt your nutrition and health in general.

uptake of Calcium and Bone Health:

Vitamin D is necessary for the uptake of calcium in the intestines, which helps seniors keep their bones healthy.

Fall Prevention:

Seniors often have a higher chance of falls, and vitamin D has been linked to muscle strength and coordination. Ensuring sufficient vitamin D levels can help to fall prevention.

Immune Support:

Vitamin D plays a part in immune system function, and seniors may benefit from immune support to reduce the risk of infections.

Mood and Cognitive Health:

Vitamin D deficiency has been linked with mood disorders and cognitive decline in seniors. Maintaining proper levels may support mental well-being.

Chronic Disease avoidance:

Vitamin D is linked to the avoidance of chronic diseases, including cardiovascular conditions and certain cancers.

Considerations for Seniors:

Sun Exposure: Vitamin D is synthesized in the skin when exposed to sunshine. Seniors, however, may spend less time outdoors. It's important to balance sun exposure for vitamin D production with considerations for skin health.

Supplementation:

Seniors may have trouble getting sufficient nutrients from food alone. Supplements may be suggested, but it's crucial to consult with a healthcare professional for personalized advice.

Medication Interactions:

Some medications widely recommended for seniors may interfere with calcium absorption or metabolism. It's important for healthcare workers to be aware of all medications and supplements being taken.

Regular Monitoring:

Regular health check-ups, including assessments of bone density and nutrient levels, can help spot and address any deficiencies or concerns.

Balanced Diet:

Encourage a well-balanced diet that includes calcium-rich foods such as dairy products, leafy veggies, and fortified foods, along with vitamin D sources like fatty fish and fortified products.

Ensuring adequate intake of calcium and vitamin D, along with other important nutrients, can significantly contribute to the overall health and well-being of seniors.

Always consult with a healthcare professional for personalized suggestions based on individual health needs.

Tips for a Bone-Healthy Diet

Maintaining bone health is important, especially as you age. A diet rich in nutrients that support bone density and strength is important. Here are some tips for a bone-healthy diet:

1. Calcium-Rich Foods:

- Include a range of calcium-rich foods in your diet. Good sources include: Dairy goods (milk, cheese, yogurt)
- Leafy green veggies (kale, broccoli, bok choy)
- Fortified plant-based milk (almond milk, soy milk)
- Tofu and fortified tofu goods

2. Vitamin D Sources:

- Vitamin D is necessary for calcium absorption. Include foods high in vitamin D:
- Fatty fish (salmon, mackerel, sardines)
- Fortified dairy or plant-based milk
- Egg yolks
- Cod liver oil
- Sunlight exposure (15-20 minutes a few times a week)

3. Protein Intake:

- Protein is important for bone health. Include healthy sources of protein:
- Fish
- Poultry
- Lean foods
- Beans and beans
- Nuts and seeds

4. Magnesium-Rich Foods:

- Magnesium is important in bone formation. Include magnesium-rich foods:
- Nuts (almonds, nuts)
- Seeds (pumpkin seeds, sunflower seeds)
- Whole grains (brown rice, quinoa)
- Leafy green veggies

5. Vitamin K Sources:

- Vitamin K is important for bone formation. Include foods high in vitamin K:
- Leafy green veggies (kale, spinach, collard greens)
- Broccoli
- Brussels sprouts

6. Phosphorus-Rich Foods:

- Phosphorus is a mineral that works with calcium for bone strength. Include phosphorus-rich foods: Dairy goods
- Meat Poultry Fish Nuts and seeds

7. Limit Caffeine and Soda:

- High caffeine intake may interfere with calcium absorption. Limit consumption of caffeinated drinks and soda.

8. Diminish Salt Admission:

- High salt admission can prompt calcium misfortune. Choose low-sodium options and limit processed and salty foods.

9. Stay Hydrated:

- Water is important for overall health, including bone health. Aim for adequate water throughout the day.

10. Balanced Diet:

- Aim for a well-balanced diet that includes a variety of food groups, providing a range of nutrients for general health.

11. Regular Exercise:

- Combine a bone-healthy diet with weight-bearing and resistance workouts to support bone strength and density.

12. Limit Alcohol:

- Excessive alcohol intake can negatively impact bone health. If you drink booze, do so in moderation.

13. Maintain a Healthy Weight:

- Being underweight or overweight can affect bone health. Strive for a healthy weight through a balanced diet and regular physical exercise.

14. Consider Supplements:

- If it's challenging to meet your nutrient needs through food alone, speak with a healthcare professional about the need for calcium, vitamin D, or other supplements.

15. Quit Smoking:

- Smoking has been linked to reduced bone density. Quitting smoking can help overall bone health.

Always speak with a healthcare professional or a registered dietitian for personalized advice based on your individual health needs and any existing conditions. They can help you build a bone-healthy diet plan that suits your specific requirements.

Lifestyle Habits to Support Bone Health

Maintaining strong and healthy bones requires more than just a balanced diet; lifestyle habits play a crucial role as well. Here are some lifestyle habits that can help bone health:

1. Regular Weight-Bearing Exercise:

Engage in weight-bearing routines such as walking, jogging, dancing, and resistance training. These activities stimulate bone formation and help keep bone density.

2. Strength Training:

Include strength training exercises to improve muscle mass and power. Strong muscles provide support to the bones and lower the risk of falls and fractures.

3. Balance and Flexibility Exercises:

Incorporate balance and flexibility exercises, such as yoga and tai chi, to improve stability and reduce the risk of falls.

4. Adequate Vitamin D Synthesis:

Spend time outdoors to allow your skin to make vitamin D through exposure to sunlight. Aim for about 15-20 minutes of sunlight on your face, arms, and legs a few times a week.

5. Limit Alcohol Consumption:

Excessive alcohol usage can negatively impact bone health. If you drink booze, do so in moderation. For adults, moderate alcohol consumption is usually defined as up to one drink per day for women and up to two drinks per day for men.

6. Quit Smoking:

Smoking has been linked to reduced bone density. Quitting smoking not only benefits your general health but also supports bone health.

7. Maintain a Healthy Weight:

Both being underweight and overweight can negatively affect bone health. Aim for a balanced weight through a combination of a healthy diet and regular physical exercise.

8. Avoid Excessive Caffeine:

While moderate caffeine intake is usually considered safe, excessive amounts can interfere with calcium absorption. Be aware of your caffeine intake, especially if you consume it in the form of caffeinated beverages.

9. Regular Health Check-ups:

Periodic check-ups can help monitor your bone density and spot any issues early on. Discuss bone health with your healthcare provider, especially if you have risk factors or worries.

10. Calcium and Vitamin D Supplementation:

If you have trouble meeting your calcium and vitamin D needs through food and sunlight alone, consult with your healthcare provider about supplements. They can suggest the proper dosage based on your individual requirements.

11. Fall Prevention Measures:

Take steps to prevent falls, as they can increase the chance of fractures, especially in older adults. This includes keeping your living area well-lit, removing tripping hazards, and using assistive devices if needed.

12. Hydration:

Stay well-hydrated as water is important for overall health, including bone health.

13. Regular Health Screenings:

Certain medical diseases, medications, and hormonal changes can affect bone health. Regular health screenings and discussions with your healthcare provider can help track and address possible concerns.

14. Dietary Considerations:

In addition to a bone-healthy diet, consider other dietary factors, such as keeping an adequate protein intake and ensuring a well-rounded nutrient profile.

15. Bone Health Education:

Stay informed about bone health and be responsible in making choices that support the well-being of your bones. Education empowers you to make informed lifestyle choices.

Remember, it's important to tailor these lifestyle habits to your individual needs and health status. Consult with your healthcare provider or a registered dietitian for personalized advice and recommendations based on your particular circumstances.

Chapter 8:

Working with Healthcare Professionals

Collaborating with Physical Therapists:

Physical therapists are experts in musculoskeletal health and play a crucial role in the control of osteoporosis. Collaborating with a physical therapist involves:

a. Assessment:

A thorough assessment of your current physical condition, including bone density, joint health, and general fitness.

Identification of specific areas of worry or weakness that need targeted attention.

b. Exercise Design:

Development of exercise plans that focus on weight-bearing and resistance training, key components for improving bone density.

Guidance on right body mechanics and posture to lower the risk of falls and fractures.

c. Lifestyle Adjustments:

Recommendations for lifestyle changes that complement your exercise program and promote overall bone health.

Integration of activities that increase bone strength into your daily life.

Communicating with Your Doctor about Exercise Plans:

Effective communication with your doctor is important for creating a personalized and safe exercise plan. This involves:

a. Health History:

Discussing your full health history, including past medical conditions, surgeries, and current medications.

Identifying any specific concerns or limitations linked to osteoporosis.

b. Goal Setting:

Clearly articulating your fitness goals, whether they involve improving bone density, general fitness, or addressing specific symptoms.

Providing your doctor with a clear idea of what you aim to achieve through your exercise plan.

c. Regular Check-ins:

Establishing a plan for regular check-ins with your doctor to monitor your progress.

Allowing for adjustments to the exercise plan based on changes in your health state or other factors.

Adapting Exercises to Health Conditions:

Osteoporosis often coexists with other health conditions, needing thoughtful adaptations to exercises:

a. Understanding Individual Health:

Recognizing and considering coexisting health conditions such as joint issues, cardiovascular worries, or balance problems.

Taking into account individual health parameters to tailor exercises properly.

b. Collaboration Between Healthcare Team:

Ensuring collaboration between physical therapists and other healthcare providers to adapt exercises properly.

Modifying intensity, length, or types of exercises based on individual capabilities and limits.

c. Variety of Exercise Options:

Exploring a variety of exercise options, including low-impact activities, aquatic exercises, or chair-based workouts, to fit specific health conditions.

Ensuring that the exercise routine stays accessible, enjoyable, and safe.

Chapter 9:

Staying Motivated

Setting Realistic Goals

Setting attainable goals is the first step in maintaining motivation in an exercise program for managing osteoporosis. This entails a multimodal strategy meant to harmonize personal capacities, goals, and states of health.

a. Realizing Personal Limitations:

Recognizing and comprehending your existing physical state is the first step towards creating attainable goals. Take into account any restrictions or health conditions related to osteoporosis, such as pain in the joints or problems with balance. This knowledge is essential for creating objectives that are safe and realistic by customizing them to your own needs.

b. Both immediate and long-term goals:

It is imperative to set a combination of short- and long-term objectives. Short-term objectives provide observable benchmarks for consistent attainment, encouraging a feeling of advancement and success. Long-term objectives, on the other hand, provide you a more comprehensive viewpoint and a feeling of direction and purpose that will keep you motivated.

c. Speaking with Medical Specialists:

Setting goals requires consulting with medical professionals, such as doctors and physical therapists. These professionals can offer insights into your physical state, assisting you in creating ambitious yet doable goals. Frequent meetings ensure continued relevance and safety by enabling adjustments based on your progress and any changes in your health status.

Choosing Pleasurable Exercises

The happiness that comes from physical activity is directly related to how long an exercise regimen can last. Finding and including fun activities improves the process's engagement and raises the possibility of long-term adherence.

a. Investigating Diverse Activities:

The best way to find out what you actually enjoy doing is to try out a range of activities. This can entail going for walks, swimming, dancing, or even participating in outdoor hobbies like gardening. Customizing your workout regimen to your tastes improves the whole experience and encourages consistency.

b. Including Hobbies:

Including hobbies in your workout regimen gives it a personalized touch. If you love music, think about working out while dancing or strolling to your preferred songs. This gives the exercise a feeling of purpose and increases enjoyment because you're fusing your favorite pastimes with fitness.

c. Group sessions and Support:

Exercise can become a social event by taking part in team activities or group sessions. The companionship of a group environment offers inspiration and encouragement. Exercise routines are more fun and lasting when people have a sense of community and are working towards similar fitness goals.

Adding Social Components to Exercise

Getting social is a great way to stay motivated during any workout regimen. Adding social components gives your program a dynamic edge and creates a nurturing atmosphere.

b. Buddy System:

Associating with a buddy or relative who has like fitness objectives establishes an internal support network. Along with accountability and mutual support, having a workout partner adds enjoyment to the program by allowing you to share experiences.

b. Group Activities:

Participating in group activities or classes fosters a sense of community and social interaction. Participating in team sports, fitness classes, or walking groups can boost motivation because of the positive energy and sense of accomplishment that is shared.

c. Online Communities:

Virtual assistance can be obtained by looking through forums or online communities devoted to osteoporosis and fitness. Making connections with people going through comparable struggles enables you to exchange advice, encouragement, and experiences. Individuals who don't have local access to group activities can particularly benefit from virtual communities.

Chapter 10:

Frequently Asked Questions

Developing a safe and efficient exercise program requires an understanding of the questions and concerns around exercise in people with osteoporosis. This chapter covers frequently asked questions, safety issues, and concerns to help people start their workout regimen with confidence.

Frequently Asked Questions Regarding Exercise and Osteoporosis

People with osteoporosis face particular difficulties, and they frequently share worries about their fitness routine. It is essential to address these issues in order to promote motivation and a sense of security.

A. Impact on Bone Wellbeing:

 "Can practice truly work on bone thickness? is the question.

It has been demonstrated that strength training and weightlifting increase bone density. A customized workout regimen helps strengthen bones and lower the chance of fractures.

b. Fracture Risk:

"Does exercise increase the risk of fractures for individuals with osteoporosis?" is the question.

In response, carefully planned workouts performed under medical professionals' supervision can strengthen bones and enhance balance, hence lowering the chance of fractures.

c. Appropriate Exercise Types:

"What kinds of exercises are safe for people with osteoporosis?"

In general, low-impact exercises such as swimming, walking, and strength training are safe. Speak with medical experts to create a plan that suits your specific requirements.

Taking Care of Safety and Pain Concerns

Every workout program should prioritize safety, and those who have osteoporosis may need to take extra precautions. By addressing these issues, a safe and injury-free approach to fitness is ensured.

a. Fall Avoidance:

"What steps could I at any point take to prevent falls while working out? Is the question.

The answer is to concentrate on workouts that improve coordination and balance. When necessary, use assistive technology, and select activities that reduce the chance of falling.

b. Torment The executives:

"How would it be advisable for me to respond in the event that I hurt while working out?

In response, pain must not be disregarded. Adjust or cease painful exercises, and seek medical advice to address any underlying problems.

c. Stance and Body mechanics:

"How significant are legitimate stance and body mechanics?" is the question.

The key to preventing injuries is to maintain good body mechanics and posture. Under a physical therapist's supervision, pick up and hone methods.

Modifying Exercises for Particular Situations

When designing an activity program, people with osteoporosis may have coexisting medical issues that need to be carefully taken into account. Exercise modifications guarantee safety and inclusion.

a. Joint difficulties:

"Is it safe for people with joint problems to exercise?"

Absolutely, workouts can be changed to account for joint problems. Exercises that improve range of motion and low impact might be advantageous.

b. Cardiovascular Issues:

"What is the impact of osteoporosis on people with cardiovascular conditions?"

Exercises can be modified to address cardiovascular issues. Creating a balanced routine requires consulting with a healthcare practitioner.

c. Balance Issues:

"What exercises are suitable for those with balance issues?" is the question.

Exercises that improve balance, such tai chi or certain stability exercises, can be included. Maintain a secure atmosphere and seek assistance when required.

Appendix:

Exercise Charts and Resources

The appendix is a useful resource that includes workout charts and useful information to help folks on their osteoporosis exercise journey. It offers sample workout regimens as well as tips on evaluating progress and modifying intensity.

Exercise Charts

Exercise Plans

a. Bone-Building Exercises:

Weight-bearing and resistance activities that specifically target bone health are illustrated in charts.

For each exercise, specific instructions on proper form and technique are provided.

b. Low-Impact Activities:

Charts outlining low-impact activities appropriate for people with osteoporosis.

Variations and adjustments to match varying levels of fitness.

c. Exercises to increase Flexibility and Balance:

Visual guidance to exercises to increase flexibility and balance.

Step-by-step recommendations for improving stability and lowering the risk of falling.

Exercise Routine Examples

a. Beginner's regimen:

- A sample fitness regimen for beginners that focuses on fundamental exercises.
- Gradual development to increase strength and fitness.

b. Intermediate Level Routine:

- A more difficult routine for people who have some workout experience.

- Included a variety of workouts to improve bone health and overall well-being.

c. Advanced Workout Plan:

- Designed for those with a greater degree of fitness.
- Dynamic workouts to maintain bone density and boost cardiovascular health are included.

Monitoring Progress and Changing Intensity

a. Progress Tracking Log:

- A log form for tracking exercise frequency, duration, and perceived intensity.
- Gives a graphical picture of progress over time.

b. Intensity Adjustment Guidelines:

- Information on how to assess and alter workout intensity.
- Tips on how to adjust intensity based on individual capabilities and goals.

c. Consultation and help Resources:

- A list of recommended resources for more assistance and help, such as books, websites, and organizations.
- How to seek professional help from healthcare providers, physical therapists, and fitness gurus.

The exercise charts and materials in this appendix are intended to empower people with osteoporosis by providing them with useful tools for their exercise program. These resources provide a thorough introduction to safe and effective exercises, sample routines, and techniques for tracking progress, whether you are a beginner or an advanced fitness level. Before beginning a new fitness program, always consult with a healthcare expert and alter activities depending on individual needs and restrictions.

Conclusion

I celebrate the transformational power of movement and its profound impact on bone health, overall well-being, and quality of life as we conclude our thorough guide on exercises for osteoporosis books for seniors. This experience has demonstrated the human body's resilience and the possibility for positive transformation, even in the face of osteoporosis. As we say goodbye to the pages of this book, consider the major lessons obtained and the route forward toward a life of strength, flexibility, and vitality.

A Comprehensive Approach to Osteoporosis Management

We have underlined the necessity of a comprehensive strategy to addressing osteoporosis in elders across these pages. It is more than just recommending specific activities; it entails cultivating a lifestyle that promotes bone health. Engaging in weight-bearing exercises, including balance and flexibility routines, eating a nutritious diet, and cultivating a positive mindset all contribute to a well-rounded osteoporosis management plan.

Knowledge Provides Empowerment

Understanding leads to empowerment, and this book aimed to offer seniors with the knowledge and skills they need to take care of their bone health. We want to empower our readers to make informed decisions about their health by revealing the secrets of osteoporosis, detailing the science underlying activities, and elucidating the link between lifestyle choices and bone density.

Strengthening and Resilience

The activities on these pages are foundational for developing strength and resilience. Weight-bearing activities like walking and strength training, as well as balance-enhancing exercises like tai chi and yoga, all play an important role in reinforcing bones, increasing muscle development, and improving general stability. The journey toward increased strength is about bolstering the spirit in order to tackle obstacles with tenacity and drive.

Promoting Community and Help

When the journey to greater health is shared, it is frequently more gratifying. This book urges seniors to seek out supportive communities, such as group exercise classes, internet forums, and local wellness clubs. Shared experiences, counsel, and encouragement can be a powerful force in conquering the obstacles of osteoporosis. Seniors can encourage and uplift one another as a community on their journey to better health.

Creating Mind-Body Balance

We have looked beyond the physical components of exercise to the profound relationship between mind and body. Mindful practices, meditation, and relaxation techniques have been identified as critical components of a comprehensive osteoporosis care strategy. Seniors can improve their overall quality of life by cultivating a sense of calm and mental well-being.

A Lifetime Journey

As we come to the end of this course, it is critical to remember that the pursuit of optimal bone health is a lifelong endeavor. It is never too late to begin, and consistency is essential. Every workout, every mindful moment, and every healthy lifestyle decision helps to lay the groundwork for a healthier, more vibrant existence. Seniors are reminded that this is a marathon, not a sprint, and that each stride forward is an accomplishment in and of itself.

Final Thoughts

As we say goodbye to these pages, we send our best wishes for a future filled with strength, resilience, and joy. May the exercises in this book serve as companions on the way to greater bone health, and may the knowledge learned provide elders with the confidence to embrace vitality and well-being. The journey to optimal bone health can be challenging, but with drive, education, and a commitment to a comprehensive approach, it can be an enriching and transformative experience. Here's to a full life full of movement, power, and the limitless possibilities that lay ahead.

Review Page

Dear Reader,

Thank you for taking the time to comment on "Exercises for Osteoporosis Book for Seniors." I appreciate your concern, and I have revised this book to make it more comprehensive and appropriate for seniors suffering from osteoporosis.

It's extremely satisfying to know that the expert advice, progressive fitness routines, and safety features sparked your interest. I see the significance of delivering activities that not only efficiently target bone health but also promote senior safety and well-being. Your praise for the user-friendly layout and motivational aspects is heartening, as I worked hard to make the book accessible and entertaining for a wide spectrum of readers.

I am dedicated to providing seniors with the information and resources they need to actively manage their osteoporosis, and your good feedback confirms that we are on the right course. Please provide any more comments, suggestions, or specific elements you'd like me to cover in future editions.

Thank you once more for your encouragement and suggestion. I am pleased that "Exercises for Osteoporosis" has had a positive impact, and I hope that it will continue to be a valuable resource for seniors looking to improve their bone health.

Best regards,

[Esther R. Johnson]